Dear Heather,
I am so grateful we
joined forces & are now
inspiring & supporting one
Im really happy you are in a
Hope you enjoy the boo—
your motivation & excit—
yours :)

How A Painful Journey With

Ps—

oriasis Became A Life Devoted To Healing Others

IT'S ALL ABOUT
LOVE

KIM WEILER

Ps—

How A Painful Journey With **Ps**oriasis Became A Life Devoted To Healing Others

IT'S ALL ABOUT
LOVE

outskirts
press

Outskirts Press, Inc.
http://www.outskirtspress.com

ISBN: 978-1-4787-7924-7

Library of Congress Control Number 2016913612

Cover Photo © 2017 thinkstockphotos.com. All rights reserved - used with permission.
Author Photo © 2017 Peter Hurley All rights reserved - used with permission.
Alkaline food chart courtesy www.phreshproducts.com

Outskirts Press and the "OP" logo are trademarks belonging to Outskirts Press, Inc.

PRINTED IN THE UNITED STATES OF AMERICA

MAX

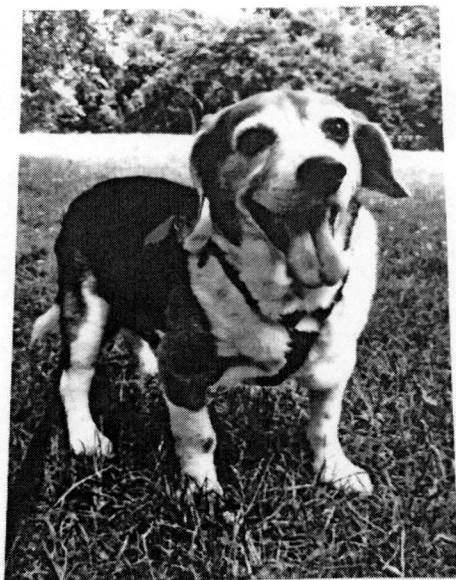

MY ADORING AND UNCONDITIONALLY LOVING TEACHER.
IT IS BECAUSE OF YOU
THAT I STARTED MY HEALING JOURNEY.

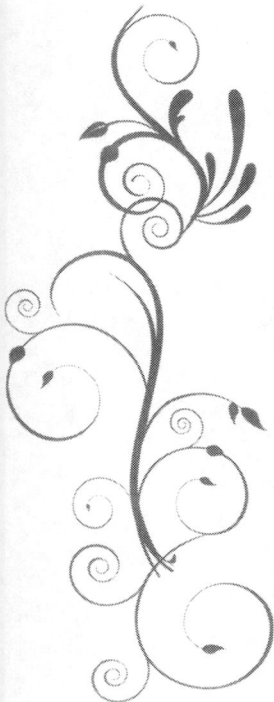

Dedication

I dedicate this book to all who have ever suffered from a skin disorder. I am here to tell you that there is hope, you can recover, and that nothing in the world is more important to me than knowing I somehow helped you start this healing journey. Fear and self-image issues have prevented you from living a full life of happiness and joy, but no more; the time to take control of your health and live life to the fullest is now.

Psoriasis (Ps): I love you.

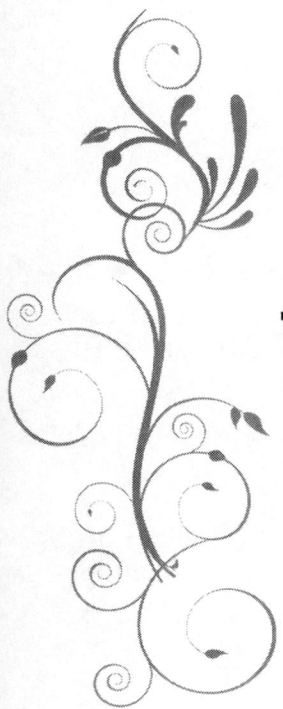

Table of Contents

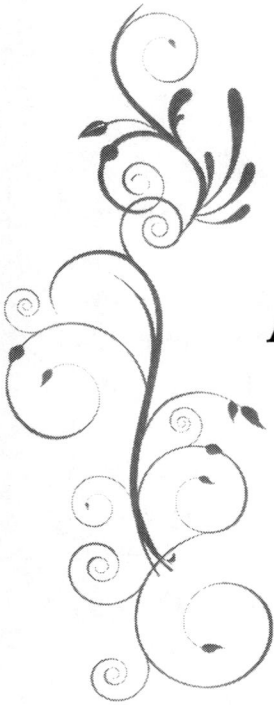

Acknowledgments

As I think about this long and exciting journey, the list of people I need to thank could be another book, but let me begin here. I could never have written this without Max, my faithful mutt, who lives on in my heart and was by far my greatest, most unconditionally loving teacher and companion.

Beyond my one physically challenged little dog who opened the door for me, I would like to thank so many others. My parents, for their loving support and teaching me the value of working hard at everything you do. My sister, Stacey — I honestly don't know what I would do without you; you are my best friend. Marley, for making me sound like a better writer than I am; I am in awe of your brilliance and beyond grateful you are in my life. Eric, who has done an excellent job of editing and helping make my dream come true. Lisa, my incredible photographer and friend. All those in my beautiful, loving friendship network who encouraged and supported me during this time and throughout various stages of my life. And, of course, my rock, my hubby Mike, for his undying love and support: thank you for listening to me talk about this book for months on end, for suffering through the bad recipes while becoming my test kitchen subject, and for always being willing to grow and learn. Our love nourishes me, empowers me, and makes me the happiest woman on the planet. To have recently become Mrs. Matullo is a feeling that no words can express. Thank you.

I also want to thank the Institute for Integrative Nutrition for teaching me that we need a self-care system more than a health-care system, and for opening up my world to primary food and how it plays a huge part in my mindful path every day.

And, lastly, to my skin: thank you for never giving up on me and making me pay attention to the fact that even I deserve self-love.

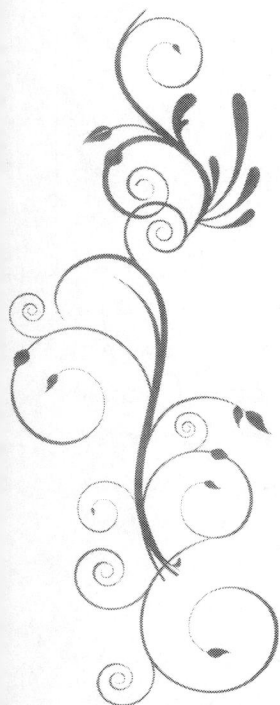

Notable Introduction and Praise for Ps - It's All About Love:

How a Painful Journey with Psoriasis Became a Life Devoted to Healing Others

If you're reading this book, chances are you or someone you know has been touched by the autoimmune disease psoriasis. This is a condition that can turn soft and smooth skin into patches of thick, white scales that become incredibly itchy and can even bleed due to excessive scratching. But it doesn't stop there; the effect this condition can have on your inner world is just as startling.

Although I've made a career out of being a Talk Show Host and Brand Spokesperson, there was a time in my life when I wasn't able to walk properly, let alone hold a job. I was diagnosed at ten years old with psoriasis and what started as a few small patches eventually covered 90% of my body. Then, about ten years into that diagnosis, my joints were affected and I developed psoriatic arthritis. At the time, I didn't even know this kind of disease existed and there wasn't a soul I knew who had it or anything similar.

I felt alone in my struggle, disappointed with my body and incredibly frustrated by my outward appearance. From the age of 10 to 25, the only thing I really knew about myself was that I was "sick." It consumed so much of my day that it was pretty much all I could think about. Whether I was anxious about the pain I would experience getting my skin wet to take a shower, or nervous about wearing dark clothes because skin flaking would make my illness visible to others, or even fearful about meeting new people because questions and suppositions on my condition would arise, I was consumed both mentally and physically.

Then, one day, something shifted within me and I have never been the same since. I was lying in bed, unable to move without severe pain and I was all alone. My parents were living in Hong Kong and I had just been through a divorce which had left me heartbroken. As I lay there, I got a call from a friend of mine asking me if I wanted to meet up with her for a fun day. She was trying to cheer me up, but I declined her invitation because I couldn't get out of bed. I hung up the phone and felt beyond frustrated with my situation. So much so, I finally decided to stop owning my struggle so fiercely. I decided to start the practice of focusing on all the beauty in my life versus all the pain; even on the days where beauty was especially hard to find. It might sound simple and maybe even insignificant to make this change, but I assure you it was not.

I had to call on the deepest parts of myself to begin reprogramming my brain to not be defeated by the way my physical body was outwardly looking and to believe in something greater than my physical circumstances. By this time, I had already done a bunch of introspective courses. I had gotten trained to be a life coach and I had read countless self-help books. But it wasn't until I was finally sick of being sick that things changed.

It's this journey, and Kim's journey, that brought us together. We both know what it's like to feel so defeated by this condition. The amazing news is this: there is a better way. Kim has outlined it all for you.

The principles and concepts that she talks about in her book are easy for anyone to use and apply. She's made her healing journey very relatable. In fact, it's something you can start implementing right now. However, you need to be ready. As I have learned over the 25 years of living with psoriasis and psoriatic arthritis, there is no quick fix for this condition and in many ways I have learned to have a deep sense of gratitude for that.

It's my belief that our bodies are our biggest teachers. They show us when we aren't aligned with something, when we are too stressed or even when we have unresolved anger festering within. But are we listening when our body is trying to get our attention? Often, we are not. So as you start this journey towards loving yourself more and walking towards true healing, are you ready to listen to your body like your life depends on it? Because chances are, it does.

Nitika Chopra
Talk Show Host and Self-Love Expert
www.NitikaChopra.com

Ps: It's all About Love is a must read. Not only is it a compassionate and inspiring portrayal of Kim Weiler's triumphant journey of healing her own psoriasis but it is an innovative comprehensive strategy that includes an easy-to-follow action plan for anyone who has exhausted the traditional methodologies for managing and curing skin diseases. Through nutrition (ironically spear-headed by her devotion to caring for her ailing dog), self-love and self-care, she shares her struggles and sheds light on how to heal through focusing on body, mind and spirit.

I wish I had this resource years ago when I suffered with psoriasis while modeling in magazines, TV and on the runway. It was a constant battle to keep my "secret" under wraps and avoid exposing my less than flawless skin patches to my agents, clients and photographers. Nutrition, self-love and self-care have been the pillars for keeping my skin clear for decades. Thank you, Kim, for sharing your insights, love and wisdom with all those who suffer from this condition and are desperately searching for a cure! I highly recommend this book to each of you!

Mary Giuseffi
Personal Brand Expert
Best Selling Author
Former Ford Model
www.marygiuseffi.com

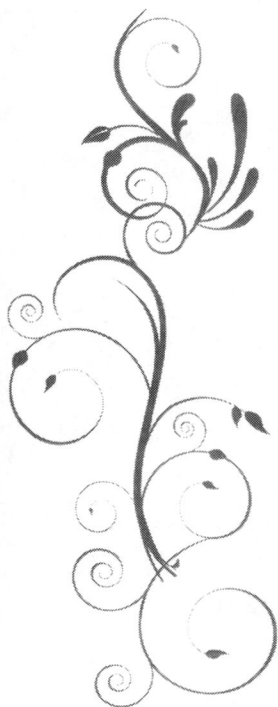

Introduction

Very few people start this journey of life saying, "I'm going to come into a body, grow up with issues, have painful memories, have a life that is wracked with guilt, illness, and pain, and then die." I certainly am not one of them. But then, I have been described as one of the most positive women others have known. Hiding under this exterior and persona, however, may have been a woman not quite as perfect as others might have imagined. Being seen as an actress, a professional, a communicator, a thinker, and a questioner of all things with a constant smile on my face could be why people see me differently than I have seen myself for years. For that reason, I am sharing my story. I feel compelled to help others and feel that, by revealing my flawed self, I can help you too. Strange to say, I feel fortunate to have been gifted with hard life lessons to prove that, through helping oneself and others, you can find a new skin to live in — both metaphorically and literally.

The new life I have found and the new being I have become could only have evolved from my undergoing some challenging experiences. And now, whether you're reading this book for yourself or a loved one, I want you to find the same joy, peace, and health that I have discovered — without having to struggle for twenty-one years, as I have. I can confidently say that I am now the happiest person I have ever been, with the deepest desire and passion to help others who struggle around me. My illness has become my mission. That is the reason I wrote this book, and that is what I believe life is all about. So, whether you start here at the beginning and dig into the answers and what I have learned, or you jump to the end to hear more about my journey and what makes me an authority on this topic, I am grateful you found me. I can't wait for a day to meet you and hear about you, your journey, and your progress. I will be here to help you in any way I can.

Joseph Campbell, who taught us so much about human nature, was correct: Isn't it time you give up that old life you planned and create the new and healed one that awaits you?

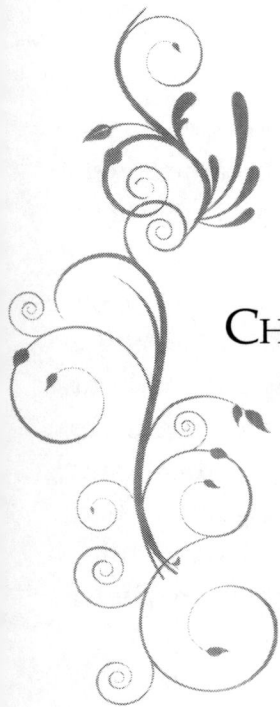

Chapter One
My Dog Saved My Life

*Do you know how many
calories are in butter and cheese
and ice cream? Would you get
your dog up in the morning for a
cup of coffee and a donut?*

Jack LaLanne

It all started with my dog, Max, who is sadly no longer with us. Long story short, Max was a rescue, and I took him in despite his slew of medical issues. His weight was always an issue, and I had been trying to get him to lose it for years, but nothing worked. He was on prescription medication for epilepsy and chronic bronchitis (COPD), took cough suppressants, used an inhaler, and had arthritis. He even took heartworm prevention medications, since he had almost previously died from that.

Yes, you read correctly, he was on all those medications, and he was on an inhaler! As much as this always shocked people and I hated using it, it worked. It was a typical inhaler a human would use for asthma, but it goes into this plastic device that has a rubber mask on the end that fits around the dog's muzzle. When you spray the drug, the dog breathes it in, and it helps relax the muscles, which in turn opens up the respiratory tract airways and allows the dog to breathe better. The process helps reduce inflammation and clears out mucus from the lungs (similar to what happens with humans).

I'd keep the mask on for as long as Max would allow, usually five seconds (if I was lucky). My vet said this was the better option because it affected his lungs directly without affecting other organs, and without Max having to experience other side effects. I was willing to try anything at this point; one of his medications for epilepsy, prednisone, already had him drinking a ton of water and peeing every twenty minutes. He was a walking, barking, medicine-taking machine, and I was the one in charge of administering all of it.

Due to his weight and poor overall health, my vet suggested I try feeding him healthy human food such as chicken, brown rice, and sweet potatoes. She said most dog food, even the most expensive, organic kind, was still processed, leftover scraps from who-knows-what or who-knows-where. Around the same time, a friend of mine, Katie Newman, was writing a book, *The Amazing Treat Diet for Dogs*, about saving her dog's life from obesity by changing his diet. She created a regimen for her dog that included vegetables and fruits. Between my vet's advice and my friend's book, in four months, my dog lost nine pounds and went from struggling to walking to outright running. To my amazement and utter thrill, most of his ailments disappeared, and he was able to be weaned off all of his medications.

Then the epiphany.

Can you imagine the moment I realized that if I could make this happen for a dog what would happen if I took the same approach for myself? I had been struggling with psoriasis for sixteen years, and it took a vet to clue me in to this possibility?

Somehow, seeing Max's miraculous recovery triggered a need to learn more about the process of eating whole foods, and I felt compelled to research and study anything I possibly could on the issue of eating to heal versus simply eating to survive. This changed my view about food altogether, because now, I saw that you really are what you eat.

At the same time that I was researching food, eating healthier, and working hard to learn about everything I was about to put in my mouth (as I share in Chapter Four, for those who need to skip ahead), I became addicted to films such as *Food Inc.*, *Food Matters*, *Hungry for Change*, *Crazy Sexy Cancer*, *The Gerson Miracle*, and *The Beautiful Truth*, just to name a few. It's amazing that, these days, we think nothing of absorbing a book (that arrived two days after you ordered it), the internet, and movies all at the same time in search of answers. Instant access means instant learning, and when you're on a mission to cure yourself, that has its benefits.

I started to juice fresh vegetables and fruits every day and gave up all meat—not just red. I started reading a lot of books written by amazing people who had healed themselves of ailments or disease. One woman whose book changed my life is Kris Carr, and the book is *Crazy Sexy Diet*. She's an amazing woman who was diagnosed with Stage IV cancer, and then beat the odds through her healthy lifestyle. I encourage everyone to read her books and take inspiration from her.

My new healthy way of eating was helping me feel better. I had tons of energy and was beyond regular (if you know what I mean). I was not only proud of myself but excited at my new physical stamina. However, after many months of this hard work, my psoriasis wasn't clearing up, and every so often I'd still find parts of me covered in those red scaly bumps. It was frustrating and confusing when all I wanted to do was to get healed.

At one point, I had a particularly large patch on my shin, and I decided to visit my dermatologist to see if there were any new creams I could try. Every time I went to see her, I'd find myself asking her about diet and the effects on my skin and what I could do to help myself get better. She'd always have the same response: she'd roll her eyes slightly and say there was no proof that diet makes any difference. She was clearly not a believer in the healing benefits of food, and I would always leave feeling a little stupid for having asked. I trusted that she had to be right because she's the doctor.

I talked to her about my extra-large patch and how stubborn it was being. She suggested laser therapy for the umpteenth time, but I didn't feel I could make the commitment of three days a week for six months. She then suggested giving the patch a shot of cortisone, promising that this would do the trick while warning me that it would be painful. When she told me that, I felt like puking. I felt gross. It felt wrong. Deep down, I knew that treating anything from the outside-in was not the answer. I had watched too many documentaries to know that food is our medicine, or at least it was years ago before it was over-processed or sprayed with chemicals. I declined the shot, left with a bunch of free samples of a new cream I couldn't afford, and felt alienated because even my doctor thought I was on the wrong track.

I came out of that appointment upset, but somehow something in me was triggered. I threw myself at my computer and felt this urge to google psoriasis. I was stunned at all the information that was out there. I wondered why I hadn't thought to google it before. Why, in sixteen years, had I never thought to do my own research about this? I still don't have an exact answer to that question, but I do believe that everything happens at the time it happens for a reason!

I researched everything, from online chat groups to YouTube videos to whatever I could find. What was most amazing to me was to find thousands and thousands of sufferers, most in worse condition than me. During my searches, I stumbled upon Dr. John O. A. Pagano's book, *Healing Psoriasis: The Natural Alternative*, which has proven invaluable to me as a source of information.[1] I also came across the site merryclinic.com, where I read, "Skin inflammation is a sign that toxins are inside your body." The second I read that, a lightbulb went off in my head, and I thought, *Now this makes perfect sense*. How interesting, right?

After reading more about their explanations of the psoriasis process, I had this enticing feeling that I was on to something. I couldn't ignore the fact that this concept of toxins in the bloodstream made so much sense to me. Not only that, my gut was feeling something I hadn't felt before: relief. I had been in the dark for so long, and now a little bit of light was being shed — and was it ever relieving!

I don't feel it was an accident I found Dr. Pagano's book. If there is such a thing as divine intervention, this was it. In the meantime, Dr. Pagano's definition of psoriasis read:

> Psoriasis is the external manifestation of the body's attempt to "throw off" internal toxins. In other words, to put it more succinctly, the skin is doing what the

---

1   Dr. John O. A. Pagano, *Healing Psoriasis: The Natural Alternative* (Hoboken, New Jersey, John Wiley & Sons, 2008).

bowels and the kidneys should be doing. The skin is not ordinarily designed to remove waste matter to any great extent, but, due to the toxic overload produced by a leaky gut, it acts as a backup system and takes on the task of removing toxins — thus the rash, irritation, and lesions. [2]

I don't know about you, but my whole body was screaming, "Yes, that makes total sense!"

Pagano explained how toxins get into the bloodstream, why that happens, and how to heal. His entire philosophy is about healing the skin from the inside through various healthy avenues, including diet, herbal teas, vitamins, a positive attitude, and internal cleansing. The book both inspired and motivated me. Before I even finished reading it, I started planning my new way of life; one that I knew would be difficult, but I was on a mission to heal my skin, and nothing would stop me. Something in me was just so done living with a skin disease.

Dr. Pagano's program has a diet that includes eating mostly alkaline, less-acidic foods. It requires staying away from foods that cause inflammation, such as red meat and most dairy. Sounds terrible, right? Want to hear the worst part? Coffee and alcohol are acidic. This was — and still is — the hardest part for me. I worked in New York City at the time and used to walk everywhere with a coffee in hand, just like 99 percent of the other New Yorkers. It completed my walk. It completed me. I can't explain the comfort in it, but it just did.

Dr. Pagano also listed a few foods to absolutely avoid because they are harmful if you have skin disorders or arthritis. The list was shocking to me as, among other things,

---

2   Pagano, *Healing Psoriasis*, 2

it includes tomatoes, eggplant, white potatoes, peppers, and paprika. These are known as the nightshades. Even worse, in addition to being a nightshade, tomatoes "carry an enzyme that is powerfully destructive to the psoriatic, eczematous, and arthritic patient." [3] (You might also be very curious to learn, and I discuss it later, that the tobacco plant is also a nightshade!)

I have since researched nightshades more and learned that they produce a natural pesticide called glycoalkaloid and a protein called lectin. Both can contribute to "leaky gut syndrome," which is a condition that most people dealing with an autoimmune disease have without even knowing it. Apparently, there are so many people with leaky gut walking around, don't be surprised if you are one of them.

Leaky gut is very much like it sounds; it's when your digestive tract develops small holes that allow certain substances or food particles to get through that usually should not. All sorts of things cause these holes to occur, such as stress, toxic medications, processed foods filled with chemicals, over-acidic foods that cause inflammation, and large food particles. These holes get bigger over time and then allow bad things to pass through, such as bad bacteria, toxic waste, and, although it doesn't sound bad, proteins such as gluten.

Because gluten is so topical, allow me to expand. Gluten is a mixture of proteins found in wheat and other grains which can cause inflammation in the intestines, and in turn, create a leaky gut. More and more people are becoming aware of their sensitivity to it. It can have serious consequences, most notably celiac disease. Other common reactions include fatigue, brain fog, diarrhea or constipation, heartburn, bloating,

---

3   Pagano, *Healing Psoriasis*, 6

vomiting, and gas. Some people with gluten intolerance can develop autoimmune skin diseases such as psoriasis, dermatitis, and eczema. Even traditional doctors and experts are now linking it to brain diseases such as Alzheimer's, dementia, and disorders such as depression.[4]

Back to the toxic waste. As a result of the leaky gut syndrome, this toxic waste can seep through your intestinal walls straight into your bloodstream, which can wreak havoc on your brain, your eyesight, your equilibrium, and…you name it. This is not a good scenario. Your immune system sees these particles or substances as foreign invaders and responds by defending itself because it doesn't recognize them and sees them as threats to your body. As a result, your body attacks itself, thus leading to food intolerances and autoimmune diseases. So, as much as you may be upset about your symptoms and how you look or feel, realize that it's a gift from your body trying to warn and protect you.[5]

It's pretty amazing what our bodies can do and how hard they work for us every day. We should be thanking them and trying to help them, not putting more damaging things in and on them.

In case you think I am scolding you, you would be so very wrong! I think back on my college days, when I studied for years at diners with friends, eating gravy fries every night at 2 a.m. It's amazing my body is even willing to help me heal at

---

4　　http://www.webmd.com/digestive-disorders/celiac-disease/news/20061013/celiac-disease-linked-dementia.

5　　Much of the information about leaky gut was derived and summarized from the following websites: Dr. Josh Axe, "4 Steps to Heal Leaky Gut and Autoimmune Disease," Dr. Axe, http://draxe.com/4-steps-to-heal-leaky-gut-and-autoimmune-disease/; Dr. Sarah Ballantyne, "The WHYs behind the Autoimmune Protocol: Nightshades," The Paleo Mom, August 22, 2012, http://www.thepaleomom.com/the-whys-behind-auto-immune-protocol/; Dr. Georgia Ede, "How Deadly Are Nightshades?" Diagnosis Diet, http://www.diagnosisdiet.com/nightshades/.

this point in my life. Nightshades were foods I ate on a daily basis. Tomatoes are still the most difficult to resist because, again, think New Yorker. Think of a New Yorker not able to indulge in famous New York pizza. Traitor! Even worse, no tomatoes means no salsa, marinara sauce, tomato-based soups, chili, ketchup, lasagna, many seasonings, veggie burgers (like it or not, tomatoes are a very common ingredient in these items) and so on. The list never ends. Tomatoes are the base for so many dishes and very hard to avoid. What was I going to eat on my pasta? What was I going to use to flavor my turkey burger other than ketchup? What's life without a gooey, yummy chicken parmigiana?

Never mind tomatoes — what's a meal when you're in college, or fresh from an acting gig and hanging with buddies, that isn't capped off by a cigarette and a walk down the avenue watching New York City hustle by? We all know smoking causes lung cancer, but the acidic effect that tobacco wreaks on your body compounds a whole slew of other conditions and illnesses. As Dr. Pagano explains, "Nightshade, as some of my readers know, is a deadly poison" and that "since tobacco is also a nightshade plant, smoking should be completely avoided, or at least greatly curtailed."[6] He then goes on to share that "about 25 percent of all psoriasis cases have their origin in smoking. In case you are wondering, secondary smoke is just as harmful as actually smoking yourself."[7] I was stunned when I read this because I started smoking back in college — thinking it was cool — and that was right around the time I developed psoriasis! Coincidence? (I share this to let you know that I've been there and hold absolutely no judgment. I just want to help you learn what may be causing your psoriasis breakouts.)

6   Pagano, *Healing Psoriasis*, 80
7   Ibid., 81

Back to food. What about white potatoes? French fries? Dipping my turkey in mashed potatoes and gravy on Thanksgiving and every wonderful holiday or party from here on in? Everything I was used to was changing, and I knew it required making a commitment. I had to be the change. But as excited as I was for the journey, little did I know how hard the process would be. A human making a change for themselves versus one being strict for a pet are two different things. Funny how we can put a dog on a specific diet (out of love) and make it stick to it, but we can find all sorts of excuses not to care for ourselves. The bottom line is, I had to change everything, and that is what I explore and share in this book.

I explore the foods, the drinks, the mess-ups, the achievements, the pain, the crazy mental games, the shifting interpersonal relationships and, most importantly, the neurotic things we do to fit in no matter how destructive they are to our well-being. I also share encouragement and strength and ways to overcome, because I've been there and want you to succeed. I want to teach you how not to suffer.

I'll leave you with this thought before diving into the meat of this book: about a year before Max died, I had taken him to get his annual checkup, and the vet was astonished. She said that Max's insides were that of a six-month-old puppy! Can you believe that? I couldn't. He was eleven and on multiple medications for epilepsy, chronic bronchitis (COPD), arthritis, and heartworm prevention. This was a dog that couldn't even walk! It still amazes me to this day.

The fact that I learned about healing from my beloved Max is a gift I will cherish forever. I am so glad he shared his life and love with me, and I hope this story will prove to you that sometimes answers come from unexpected places, so always be aware. You never know where a wonderful lesson may come from.

Ps: I love you, Max!

Meditation

Think of something you are grateful for right now. Now, think of something hard, a challenge, a loss, an illness that happened or is happening in your life. Thank it for having come into your body, your life, and bless it by telling it how much it meant, but now tell it that it is time to go. Feel love and warmth all around you because you know that you are saying goodbye to that season and hello to a new, healthier one. While you meditate, and throughout the day, know that I am with you on this journey, and know that you are loved.

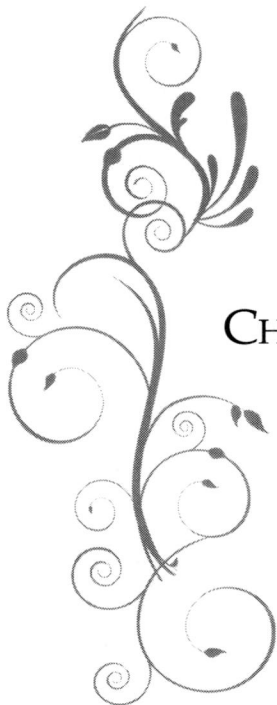

CHAPTER TWO
What Is This Skin Disease, Psoriasis?

The more I learn, the more I realize I don't know.

Albert Einstein

As of writing this, I have come across 359 books, 61 academic journals, 227 magazine articles, and 1,829 newspaper articles on psoriasis (a.k.a., Ps). Does that qualify me to write a book that will help people heal?

First, the truth is, if I had realized at the outset that there was this much information available on the topic, I would have probably scared myself out of writing this book. Second, with so much information out there, why is there not a cure? Third, what have I learned that knocks just about every one of these sources off the list of what can help you?

Let me begin by saying that there is a ton of valuable information in a lot of these materials and, here in this book, I have tried to extract the absolute best and most relevant that will help chronic sufferers of psoriasis. I want to save the people who read this book from having to be the researcher that I was. I want you to skip straight to the healing and to be able to do what the universe and your soul intends for you.

(But, in case you, too, want to read everything you can about your condition, the bibliography includes all the books, movies, websites, articles, and sources that helped me the most. I am especially fond of the holistic guides and sources because they were the ones that turned my fate for the better.)

Believe it or not, before the internet made all knowledge available at a glance, people (like me) would consult encyclopedias. For example, in 2005, in Volume 12 of the *Encyclopedia of Family Health*, psoriasis is listed as a psychosomatic problem.[8] What does that mean? It means that these doctors felt it was partly a physical and partly a mental disease. I will get into this in more detail later, but for now, here's a section of an article I came across during my research:

> Psychosomatic disease mirrors those illnesses whose evolutions are channeled by psychological (thoughts, emotions, and behavior) issues; in contrast, somatopsychic diseases echo those where the biologic aspect of the disease affects the psyche. Psychocutaneous medicine impacts on the interaction between the mind, the brain, and the skin…. Factors of a psychopathological nature tend to play an etiological role in the development of skin disorders, can exacerbate pre-existing skin disorder as well as patients suffering from dermatological disorders may bear the brunt of disfigurement. Psoriasis being a key disease in the cluster of psychocutaneous disorders, it has become a focus for exploration. Due to the intimate interplay between psychosocial factors and psoriasis, this disease confirms the said definitions.[9]

---

8   David B. Jacoby and Robert M. Youngson, *Encyclopedia of Family Health*, 3rd ed., vol. 12 (New York: Marshall Cavendish, 2005).

9   "Psychosomatic paradigms in psoriasis: Psoriasis, stress and mental health," T. S. Sathyanarayana Rao, K. H. Basavaraj, and Keya Das. *Indian Journal of Psychiatry*, 2013 Oct-Dec; 55(4): 313–315.

Did they lose you? I should think so. Exactly how much in that paragraph do you think will help you heal? Isn't it wonderful that these authors, and physicians, and researchers are so very knowledgeable, but don't actually help us in our day-to-day efforts to walk out of the house psoriasis-free?

A little technical but interesting tidbit is that the word psychosomatic is from the Greek words psyche and soma. Psyche is related to the mind, and soma means body. Therefore, what I will be looking at is how much psoriasis — for which there has not been an accepted cure as of yet — is a physical reaction, and how much of it is a response to emotional issues.

What I find fascinating is that most people now understand that there is a psychological component to this condition. (I like to be positive and don't want to call it that "dis-ease" word.) Still, in the Merck Manual (the bible for physicians and pharmaceutical companies) they state:

> Psoriasis is an inflammatory disease that manifests most commonly as well-circumscribed, erythematous papules and plaques covered with silvery scales. Multiple factors contribute, including genetics. Common triggers include trauma, infection, and certain drugs. Symptoms are usually minimal, but mild to severe itching may occur. Cosmetic implications may be major. Some people develop severe disease with painful arthritis. Diagnosis is based on appearance and distribution of lesions. Treatment can include emollients, vitamin D analogs, topical retinoids, tar, anthralin, corticosteroids, phototherapy, and, when severe, methotrexate, oral retinoids, immunomodulatory agents (biologics), or immunosuppressants.[10]

---

10   "Psoriasis," Peter C. Schalock, MD, Merck Manual, http://www.merckmanuals.com/ professional/dermatologic-disorders/psoriasis-and-scaling-diseases/psoriasis.

How is it that there is not one mention of the psychological components attached to this condition? Or the mention that food, environment, and toxins can contribute to it getting worse? I could give you a long answer about pharmaceutical companies and doctor conspiracies, but I will leave it at this: after sixteen years, I started to heal only after a veterinarian opened my eyes to holistic methods and I started actively managing what I was putting in my body, not on my body.

What I will tell you — and I'm sure if you are reading this book, you know already — is that psoriasis is not contagious. I shouldn't even need to write this, but it's true. Sadly, some of my worst days and fears were related to how I thought people would respond to me and how some even did. When you are younger and in such a moldable and sensitive stage, you take everything personally, even when the person responding to you may not be educated or know better. They may simply be curious and not intend to be judgmental. Their fear of "catching what you have" could be nothing more than ignorance. But, it adds up, the weight of having to explain and of having to allay other people's fears of being around you. You're not a leper, but the comparison isn't that far off.

Then, as you age, you get more (pardon the pun) thick-skinned, and when someone asks you about your skin, you just explain it and move on. But, deep down inside, you're never free of that old fear of people judging you, of assuming they inevitably will. It remains rooted in your psyche and thoughts. For me, it wasn't the actual lesions that hurt me; it was the fear of being judged by others if they saw them.

Putting all the research and medical information together, I want to share the technical information I found the most helpful as I raced through the traditional and holistic material out there. This is the information I relate to the most these days. I learned that, along with being an autoimmune condition, psoriasis can be hereditary. I also learned that, while a normal person's skin sheds once a month when their cells mature, psoriasis sufferers endure swaths of their skin shedding rapidly every few days without the cells having a chance to mature. The cells are shedding faster than the body can handle. The result is layers of red, thick, scaly patches on your body that are incessantly itchy (and feel downright unattractive).

Dr. Mark Hyman, founder and medical director of the UltraWellness Center and chairperson of the Institute for Functional Medicine, explains autoimmunity well:

> Autoimmunity occurs when your immune system gets confused and your own tissue gets caught in the crossfire. Your body is designed to fight off harmful things like infections, toxins, allergens, or a stress response. Sometimes and for reasons not fully known, that immune army directs its hostile attack on your joints, brain, skin, and sometimes your whole body.[11]

I realized when reading his blog and understanding the complexity of the condition that my body was working overtime to heal itself. It wasn't not trying, and therefore causing these reactions that others could see; it was rapidly turning itself over because it was confused, or had a wrong signal somewhere. I realized that if, like Max, I helped my body by watching what I put into it, as well as on and around my skin, I might have a fighting chance of getting healed.

---

11 "10 Steps to Reverse Autoimmune Disease," Dr. Mark Hyman, blog, http://drhyman. com/blog/2015/09/04/10-steps-to-reverse-autoimmune-disease/.

So, if nothing else, I want you to try to love yourself enough to keep an open mind as you read through the foods, the toxins, the emotions, people's responses, and everything else we do to ourselves that makes Ps hard to heal.

I also want to share a valuable statistic: among the sufferers of the ten or so recognized types of skin conditions (eczema, acne, scleroderma, etc.), there are over 125 million people suffering from psoriasis alone. Doesn't that tell you something is wrong with the way that we are living? Doesn't that break your heart enough to want to help others? It does mine. Whatever you can do to share healing, know that it will come back to help you heal — because I do believe the positive we put out boomerangs into the positive we get back. Also, don't forget to mark your calendars every year to celebrate October 29, World Psoriasis Day. We can all join and stand strong to support each other for a cure.

In the end, I want you to know you are not alone. There are so many wonderful, supportive, positive, and knowledgeable people out there who can help you that I leave you with this thought: Today is the first day of my life, so what is the one thing I can do today to find and invite positive people into my life and move away from the negativity of others? I am not a statistic. I am me, and I know I will be healed. Whatever you want to call the condition, I want you to override any negative psoriasis connotations, call up positive buzzwords and say to yourself, "Psoriasis (Ps): I love you!"

🖎

Ps: By the way, you just took one positive step by reading this chapter.

Meditation

It's time to take back your life and your health, and I know you've got this. Just remember to keep an open mind. Think of something negative that you thought about today, or that is consuming you right now. Now, think of how to change that to a positive. For example: Although I suffer from this condition, I am getting healthy now, step-by-step. Because of my efforts, I know I will live a much longer, happier, medicine-free life as I age. Know that you, too, have the ability and will find the courage to heal yourself. Just take the first step.

Ps: I love you!

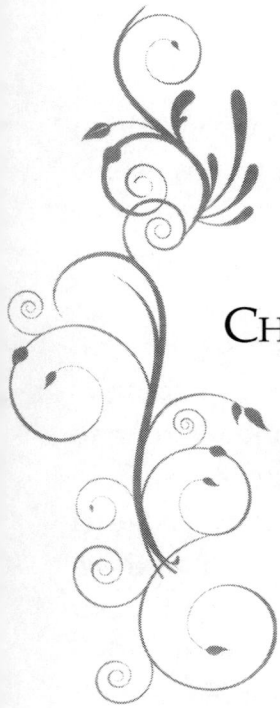

Chapter Three

"So, How Does That Make You Feel?"

The easiest time to cure an
illness is before it is accepted as
a part of the self-image.

Jane Roberts

A running but true joke for anyone who has ever been in therapy or seen a therapist interaction on TV is that you will hear them say, "So, how does that make you feel?" How does it make me feel? It makes me want to jump out of my skin, inhabit a model's body and forget about being tortured on a daily basis by the way people look at me or how I look at myself. But, since body swapping is not possible (yet), here's what I can tell you; having lesions on your body sets up all sorts of emotional reactions and causes all sorts of interferences throughout the day, whether it is with relationships, strangers, professionals, or simply making plans to go out to eat or do anything.

Let me share a few personal stories that should help you grasp what living with Ps means (which, if you're a sufferer, you'll know). Not only are these stories about what it is like to deal with Ps and the length sufferers go through to hide their condition, they are also about the amazing revelations people have had around me when they've experienced a few days or months with something on their skin that is visible to the rest of the world.

It is true that until you experience something similar, you don't know the battles a person goes through. I am going to share little stories of how we have to keep our mind strong so that we can win the battle over our chronic body issues.

People who suffer from chronic illness with no external physical symptoms struggle with different issues than those whose lesions or conditions are there for others to see. I'm not saying this is better or worse, because whether a condition or illness is visible or not, each has a different set of burdens. What I am saying is that people treat you differently up-front and immediately if they see something suspicious on the surface. If you suffer from an illness that has no signs, it's not until you share your diagnosis (or your body degenerates to the point where the illness is visible) that people then have a reaction.

If you are like me, and the lesions were visible, you did everything in your power to remain covered up because people would make comments, or say nothing yet act differently. And everywhere you went, everything you did, it came with you as if it was another part of yourself—and not the good one. It nagged at you, proving it had the upper hand. Even if you forgot, temporarily, or pretended it didn't matter, it was the unspoken elephant in the room.

A running theme in my personal life was spending hours obsessing over the fact that any man who knew about or saw my Ps would not want to date me or be with me in any way.

I felt like they would take one look and be, like, "I'm outta here." I didn't believe I'd ever find a man who would be understanding, love me for me, and not care that I had this ugly condition. I was incredibly fearful of being intimate because I never shared it up front with them. So the entire time, I was self-conscious worrying they would accidentally feel it. I even went to extreme lengths to get myself into positions where they couldn't feel or see it because, in my mind, they would be as disgusted by it as I was and not want to date me anymore.

One of my defense mechanisms was trying to convince myself that if I could just make the Ps invisible, then life would be fine, and I could find love. This way of thinking is so detrimental to one's being that it affects everything you do and places you in a position to hold secrets. Secrets you may not have had to hide in the first place. I used to do everything to hide or get rid of the Ps as quickly as possible because, like I said, if a date saw or felt it, they would ask what it was— and if they knew what it was, they would dump me. These were the thoughts in my head that could override any feelings from my heart. I couldn't believe any other human could love me with these things on my body. All I knew was that I had better get rid of it quickly before anyone found out, or I would never be loved or successful in this lifetime.

And if you think those thoughts just came and went quickly, you would be very wrong. When this type of negative thinking takes hold, anyone with an imperfection will hold on to it, repeat it, and obsess over how it is ruining their life, all the while forgetting that it is the thought that may be more of a problem than they realize. I will talk about this more in Chapter Nine on emotions and psychology, but for now, it is why I need you to turn negative statements into positives as quickly as you think of them. It doesn't matter if you buy into my process yet. It doesn't matter what you believe. It matters that you do it no matter how simple and ridiculous it sounds. This is the start of opening up. This is the start to getting rid of the baggage and negative thinking that is holding you down, whether you realize it or not. This is the start of getting rid of the things you have been hiding.

Speaking of hiding things, I want to tell you some funny stories so you can relate to the fact that we have all been there. I joke that if we had a convention of Ps sufferers we could have an entire day of meetings on the lengths people will go to hide this condition from others.

For me, there is no end to the things I have tried: the tanning salon, Revlon cover-up liquid foundation (which doesn't work), wearing long-sleeved shirts—anything and everything. I would scrub and scrub and scrub with pumice stones that are meant for your feet, thinking that the Ps would be burned off, hoping that not only would people think it was a burn, but that (deep down, hoping) it wouldn't come back in that spot. Of course, scrubbing it with anything only irritates it and makes it come back worse. I was so desperate, I was just plain stupid. All this so people wouldn't see what I was suffering from or, worse yet, comment on it.

The truth is, you can't hide it, especially once you start falling in love. And you can't live a free and fulfilling life with secrets this big. People who suffer from Ps often come from a family of secrets or things they feel they need to hide or protect. The amazing thing is that some of these secrets are known and obvious to the outside world, yet we have developed this fear around them and hold on to the secrets for dear life, regardless. I will talk more about this in my chapter on emotions. The bottom line is that you don't want to start off any relationship with lies, which is what I did when I would pretend the Ps didn't exist. Even more importantly, you can't live your life pulling away every time your lover goes to rub your arm or massage your leg.

My story of falling in love and its effect on my Ps is a bit unusual because, previous to meeting this special man, I had spent almost a year eating a plant-based diet, acidic-free for the most part, and had healed 95 percent of my Ps. Then I met my love, Mike. And I did what most people do when they start a new relationship; I sent in the representative I thought he wanted, not the real me. I started to drink and socialize more, eat more desserts after romantic dinners, and just lie to myself about the fact that I had Ps at all by acting like I could do what everyone else does.

As you can imagine, I started on a downward acidic spiral, quickly. At first, I didn't care so much because my Ps was in remission and I felt invincible. Then, we went on vacation to Ireland, and meat temporarily made its way back into my world. Of course, soon after, it all caught up with me, and my psoriasis-free elbows were no longer clear. My inner world fell apart, and I was dealt another setback. The experience I had had of walking around proud to expose my elbows when I was Ps-free had been amazing. I was shame-free, I was proud, I felt good, I looked good, and it was like nothing else in the world. It was as if I had been freed from my Ps prison, but now the gates had come crashing down on me again. It didn't help that I knew I was responsible for my own demise because I hadn't had enough strength to stick with the program that I knew had healed me.

And now, only a short while into this new relationship, with a person I knew I really cared about, all I was left with was disappointment and frustration with my situation and a constant lingering and painful feeling of being upset with myself. I knew I could do better, even knew what I needed to do, but didn't do it. And, although I am not one to ask "Why me?" or to be "Woe is me," I felt hurt and targeted, as though I was a loser. I hate that word, loser, and try never to use it, but I did feel like I had lost.

Even more fascinating, though, was that the Ps had silently crept back up on me without my even really being the first to notice. It was Mike who first noticed it, and when he did, my embarrassment was remarkable. It went like this: One night, Mike was rubbing my arms while watching TV, when he said, "What's that on your elbows, is that psoriasis?" I had no choice but to own it, look at him, and say, "Yes, yes it is." I know there could be worse moments, but that one was crappy for me. He knew I had Ps because I had told him all about my health journey when we met; but now, there he was, feeling it on my skin. That's a different story. It just made me feel so ugly, and deep down I didn't want him ever to feel that it makes me ugly because we all have imperfections and Ps does not make one ugly. My fears were so wrapped up in self-worth and appearance and putting on a face for the public that I had no idea what I was doing to myself.

The truth was, it was real. It was on my elbows, and visible, and touchable, and he had caught me. I couldn't hide it. Nor did I want to—not from him. As ashamed as I felt, I didn't want to hide anything from him. When I explained how far off my health path I'd strayed, he was so sweet; he tried to take the blame. I knew it was all my own doing, but his acknowledgment and willingness to take the blame are reasons why I fell in love with him. The good news is that this was a turning point for us. It turned out that he wanted to eat healthier as well. So, with my acknowledgment of what had happened, and knowing that the wrong food and drink can hurt our bodies, he has benefited and is now loving my positive and healthy lifestyle influence.

So, what do you do when you fall off the wagon and allow the stress of life, new relationships, or new settings get in the way? My recommendation is to start back slowly, one step at a time, one healthy meal at a time, one committed food change at a time. No doubt it will be hard. Who wouldn't be envious of going for dinner, having a few glasses of wine, and sharing a super-sugary dessert? Who doesn't want to grab a pizza when you have no time to prepare a healthy and slow dinner? Who doesn't want to eat where their friends eat and consume whatever they feel like at whatever time? It all seems so insurmountable, but it's not.

🐧

Now, I want to share with you a fascinating moment of revelation I had when a "healthy" person close to me had to deal with a condition that suddenly became visible to the world and the emotional impact it had on him. Mike had a cold sore this past winter, and that cold sore became a great lesson-learner. Remember what I said in Chapter One? Always be aware. You never know where a wonderful lesson may come from. Well, this cold sore reminds me of that.

Mike is a healthy guy, pretty secure, and kind and considerate. He's pretty normal, in a good way, and doesn't let things get to him — well, except traffic! The funny thing is that I have never seen him feel and act so insecure except for during this incident. The blessing is that, through this experience, he told me that, for the first time, he could feel himself in my shoes. He had never quite felt this feeling of shame before, having to face the world with this big, ugly sore on his lip. It was such a big deal for him, and quite a foreign feeling to him. Even though it wasn't Ps, he could finally understand the constant shame and fear of judgment. He felt uncomfortable in his skin for the very first time in his life.

While talking about this with him, I realized I had spent more of my life feeling uncomfortable in my skin than not. How is it that I had never really realized the extent of it before? It was such a learning moment for me because Mike reminded me of myself five years previous, at the beginning of my journey. He wanted answers and was on a mission to find out the cause behind this horrible feeling he had deep inside of him. He asked every friend and co-worker he knew who had gotten cold sores about their experiences. He wanted to know why he had this thing, what it is, why it develops. He felt so judged, even though no one said anything negative to his face. In Mike's head, he believed people looked at cold sores as a gross and dirty thing, probably because they are usually caused by the herpes virus. He was living in this "Why me?" mentality, feeling very helpless. It didn't help that he spent $75 on three tubes of an over-the-counter topical cream without it making any difference whatsoever. He kept filling himself up with hope only to be let down each time.

Does this sound familiar to all of you out there who have a skin disease? Watching him go nuts for almost three weeks trying anything and everything to quickly find a way to get rid of it was all too familiar. I had done it all, of course: seen the dermatologists, tried the medicinal ointments and creams, read the books, watched the movies, searched the internet. You name it, I've tried it. And now I was watching Mike do it, even though I knew, deep down, his cold sore was a result of working insane hours of overtime over the holidays and from his body being stressed out. He wasn't getting enough sleep, or exercising regularly, or eating well most of the time. His body was talking to him, saying, "Please take care of me." It was a nudge from the universe and his body that it was time to start paying attention and loving himself enough to slow down and care for the beautiful body he had been given.

His issues reminded me of the pain I used to feel and the days I used to sit in the bathroom and cry my eyes out, begging the universe to tell me why. I'd just sob because I couldn't handle the feeling of shame anymore. There was nothing left to do but cry. I was so frustrated that nothing I ever did was working. I understood very well what Mike was going through, and reassured him that it would be over soon and to let the virus take its course.

I also couldn't help with anything other than to be reassuring, and that is hard when you are the type to want to jump in and heal everyone and everything that is ailing around you. The best I could do was remind him how lucky he was that it was temporary. Perhaps not the most loving response, but I'm human, and there was the fact that, like a cold, his sore would soon be gone.

I also had odd reactions. While he felt so incredibly exposed with it being on his face, conversely, I felt lucky I could wear pants or a long-sleeved shirt to cover my skin if I needed to. I was judging him, just as I had judged myself, just as I feared others judging me. And, although the cold sore didn't bother me in some ways, it did show me how we seem to have a need to find people who are worse off than ourselves to make ourselves feel better — a human psychological trait none of us should feel proud of, but one which (if we're honest) we all exhibit.

There are a lot of people out there in this world—some I know very well—who have Ps and other skin conditions on their faces, ears, hairlines, etc. One friend of mine gets eczema on his nose and chin, and another has rosacea on her cheeks. A lot of people get dermatitis on their faces. So many people have to face the world with a low self-esteem and self-worth because of their skin conditions. It starts to define who you are that day and every day, and somehow you have to work through the feelings and the head games that make you feel worthless, or not worthy of love because you are not perfect on the outside. That's why I call Mike's cold sore my friend, my teacher. I don't think for a second we were meant to live with these conditions. Do you? That is why I feel that conflict and challenges arise to teach us a lesson. I never listened to my body before, and it took almost twenty years for me to learn that lesson.

I can tell you unequivocally, now, that when my Ps flares up, I always listen to my body for the answer. Usually, it's stress from working myself into the ground, or not making my health a priority. Sometimes it's lapsing into a poor diet because I'm only human and I really wanted that brownie. No matter what, it is a warning to pay attention and an an-nouncement that our body loves us enough to point it out.

I do want to share that the one thing I noticed the most was the sense of relief and comfort I felt when Mike told me how he understood what I must feel living with Ps. I realized how alone I had felt on this journey. It's lonely in a skin that brings you fear and shame. The fear of judgment was deep-rooted in me, and it took time and effort to release some of that. Even now, when I have a small spot appear out of nowhere, I get sucked back into that fear, and I have to remind myself it's okay, that I just need to take a deeper look at what's going on inside me. I can take control, and I can heal it. I can't be a slave to the mind games, and I must forge ahead.

Although it was only a brief period that Mike suffered, he learned to relate just a little bit more to my journey. There was comfort in that and a revelation of realizing exactly how alone I've felt. It's funny because I joke about having too many people in my life. I have a lot of wonderful friends I keep in touch with from every job I've ever had, but no matter how many loving people surround me, I'm still alone in this skin.

My journey has taught me to give myself the love I need because no matter how much I get from others, it won't be enough. I'm alone in this skin and the only way it can get the love and care it needs is from me. The love comes from letting go of the mind games that trick us into believing that we are less than perfect and, therefore, that we can never be loved, accepted, admired, or successful. We have to release the negative and let ourselves love without all the judgment.

If you were raised in an environment where unconditional love for yourself and others was ever-present and had a different form of confidence ingrained in you, there is a good chance you don't have Ps. Some people may be upset at this statement and reject it because, traditionally, doctors have told us this is a systemic or auto-immune disease, but I am here to tell you it's more. There is an emotional component.

I craved this constant feeling of comfort and acceptance of my skin, and still do to some extent, but it really hangs on us emotionally. When we don't have issues with something, we take it for granted, don't we? Sometimes we even forget about what we just went through, and that giving ourselves a break with imperfections is something we all need to work on and keep in mind. We need to remember to acknowledge and love the progress we have made, no matter how little. And if we slip up, well, acknowledge that we love ourselves enough to get back up and try again.

Acceptance of ourselves and our situations, in full-color good and bad glory, is the hardest thing to find within ourselves, especially living in a society where we are so judged by our appearance. I think the key here is, in those times where you feel your worst or feel judged the most, you need to love yourself more than ever, and never abandon yourself. You need to tell the image in the mirror that you are beautiful and worthy of love. You can't let the flawed image you may temporarily see eat at your mind. You must imagine yourself healed. You must imagine yourself whole. Because that image is the one that will become your reality in time.

My biggest piece of advice is that from this point on, you do not claim the illness, you claim that you are healed of the illness, and therefore it is only a condition that is being passed through your system at this moment and that it is on its way out. As the inspirational Jane Roberts quote says, "The easiest time to cure an illness is before it is accepted as a part of the self-image." And remember, I'm also here to help you uncover it, break free of it, and move into a whole new and wonderful life where your condition does not control you. So, try your best as you read through this book to remain open and patient. After all, it could save your skin *and* your life.

❧

Ps: Let me be your mirror for a minute and say (insert your name), I love you.

Meditation

From this point on, you do not claim the illness, you claim that you are healed of the illness, and therefore it is only a condition that is being passed through your system at this moment and that it is on its way out. Don't accept illness or conditions as part of your self-image, and do not allow yourself to play the mind games that control you or your healing by feeding yourself negative and judgmental words. You are in charge; you can win; you will be healed. That's it. Only positive thinking from here on out. Now, tell yourself you love you and read on!

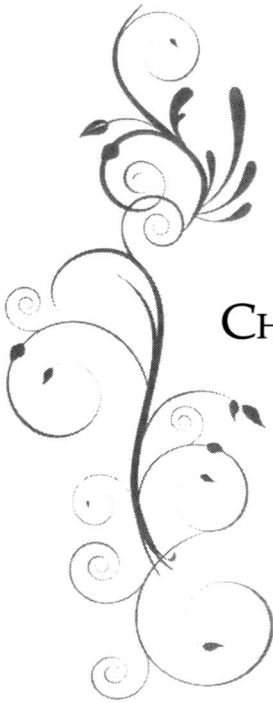

CHAPTER FOUR
Alkaline vs. Acidic

Let food be thy medicine and
medicine be thy food.

Hippocrates

How is it that the Hippocratic Oath to "first do not harm" has gone so far from the basics of what helps a human body heal? Can you believe that it was Hippocrates himself who said, "Let food be thy medicine and medicine be thy food"? What happened to us that we moved so far from the core of what nurtures us into such a processed life?

On the day that I walked out of my dermatologist's office and realized that I was pretty much alone in this journey, my destiny changed. I realized that, without a doubt, I had to be the one to take charge of my health and my psoriasis. I was not getting answers from physicians, and I had to do something.

From my mad-scientist googling, internet sourcing, movie watching, and gathering any information I could on what was out there for Ps sufferers, I made a decision early on, even before reading through all the new material, that I would start eating more alkaline foods no matter what. I had been convinced by reading the holistic materials of Dr. Pagano and others that Ps was not a skin disease as doctors claimed, but a reaction to what we put in our bodies. Funny, when you think about it, that we should go to a dermatologist — yes, a skin doctor — for something that has to do with our gut and our immune systems.

With that specific revelation in mind and because it was reverberating at a deeper level in me, I set out to make myself aware of what alkaline foods were and why they are healthier for us than acidic foods. I was a novice, as you may be — and you are not alone. To this day, anytime I mention my new alkaline lifestyle to people, the first thing they ask me is, "What are alkaline foods?" Like many people who take responsibility for what they put in their bodies, I knew some core basics: processed food is full of chemicals for preservation; red meat and dairy aren't meant to be digested by the human body, and they have been proven to cause inflammation (which causes disease); there is no point in eating fruits and veggies that have been sprayed with pesticides and chemicals; and go organic whenever possible. That's what I knew!

In America, especially, we are raised with that good old USDA food pyramid. You know, the one that says you need to use fats, oils, and sugars sparingly, but have 2-3 servings of milk, yogurt, and dairy, 2-3 servings of meat, poultry, fish, dry beans, eggs, or nuts, 3 servings of vegetables, 2-4 servings of fruit, and 6-11 servings of bread, cereal, rice and pasta … daily! Yes, you read that correctly: 6-11 servings of bread, cereal, rice, and pasta daily. And we wonder why we are facing an obesity epidemic in the United States! It's amazing that there are still people out there today who go by this chart and think it's healthy.

Therefore, learning about what is called an "alkaline versus an acidic diet" was all new to me. Let me walk you through some basics. Simply put, living an alkaline lifestyle is when you follow a more plant-based diet. What is a plant-based diet? That was the first question I had. Do I just eat plants? Fruits and veggies? I can't live on that, can I? Who can? It turns out that it's not just that, it's a whole lot more: it's fruits, veggies, various grains, seeds, nuts, legumes, herbs, and assorted spices.

Dr. Pagano recommends we consume 80 percent alkaline foods and 20 percent acidic foods. When I first started reading from his list of foods, it didn't seem all that daunting. Of course, you might feel differently. Who wants to deprive themselves of anything, right? We all know that's why any diet is such a struggle — because it means deprivation! I looked at the list of alkaline foods and thought, *Oh, a challenge, but I got this.* I was so motivated at first. But, what I wasn't thinking about was how hard it would be not to eat cheese, or drink coffee, or have a quick slice of pizza on the go if I needed to. Those thoughts never entered my mind up-front because my intention was to heal my skin and stop the feeling of shame dead in its tracks.

I learned that to understand the value and purpose of eating alkaline versus acidic food you need first to understand how your pH (acid versus alkaline) level works so that you can understand why disease can thrive in your body. An alkaline system is a growing and healing body, whereas an acidic system is a degenerating and dying body. As a visual aid, think of a basil plant that is healthy and vibrant and green and the leaves are just perfectly luscious. Now think of it when it hasn't been watered and is wilting and dry and browning and almost dead.

Give that basil plant some good watering and, bam, it comes back to life. Keep it dry and, poof, it's dead. I don't know about you, but I have seen some basil plants that looked dead come back the next day. So I want to encourage you to think positively and realize that your body wants to come back to health just as much as that little plant does, and that with a little help, it will flourish and even thrive for you.

Paraphrasing many authors on the alkaline versus acidic topic, your body's pH will come into balance by consuming a higher volume of alkaline foods. Our pH is the measure of exactly how acidic or alkaline our systems are, and this affects the growth and death of our cells. A pH of 0 is completely acidic, and a pH of 14 completely alkaline. A pH of 7 is neutral. Also, I learned that we don't just have one pH level. Our stomach has a different pH range because that's where we break down food and, therefore, it ranges from 1.35 to 3.5. It needs to be more acidic to aid in digestion. I somewhat remember learning about this in biology class in high school, but it never really meant anything to me, until now. Blood, on the other hand, must always be slightly alkaline, with an ideal pH of 7.3 to 7.5. In essence, whether or not you understand the underlying biology, you want your pH to be as close to 7 as you can manage and to push it if possible to become more alkaline. Even if you don't understand why, whatever testing method you are using, you want to move into an alkaline state.

In case you are thinking, *That's all fine, but I can't afford to go to a doctor every time I need my pH levels checked,* you can buy pH strips for use at home—and no, you don't even have to puncture yourself for blood. They come in strips for saliva and urine and are pretty inexpensive. I have purchased all different brands over the years, but right now I have some from both SelpHbalance and Phinex Diagnostic.[12] There are a bunch of brands to choose from, and most are easy to use and give a relatively accurate reading.

I have to say that it's sort of a fun game using these. I always aim to get a slightly less alkaline result than I should be aiming for because it would challenge me to eat more alkaline the next day. That being said, the days I did get good bright green results telling me that I had achieved a more alkaline state, I was super proud of myself. It kind of reassured me that I was doing well and was on the right track. If any of you use a fitness device or app, you'll know the feeling. You, too, will become a testing fiend when you get on a roll and see how valuable this knowledge is for you!

For those of you who want to understand this process better, I found a wonderful explanation of balancing pH, using strips, and exactly how our bodies work in a video online called *Acid Alkaline Balance*, by Barbara O'Neill.[13] Some of us need more information than others before they can start a new journey, and that is just fine. Others just dive in and figure it out later. No matter who you are, I honor your style of healing and just want to give you all the resources I can to help you.

A great blog called Alkaline Sisters says that "an alkaline balanced body is healthy, vibrant, and energetic, free of sickness and disease. An acidic body is one that is degenerating, breaking down, showing symptoms of ill health, from the simplest form being a cold, all the way to diabetes, heart disease, and cancer."[14] People who eat a lot of meat, dairy, sugars, alcohol, saturated fats, highly processed foods, and caffeine

---

12 SelpHbalance: http://www.selphbalance.com; Phinex: https://www.amazon.ca/Phinex-Diagnostic-Results-Seconds-Balance/dp/B003PDB79W.
13 Barbara O'Neill, "Acid Alkaline Balance": https://youtu.be/BBl1QDag2-8.
14 Alkaline Sisters: http://www.alkalinesisters.com/alkalizing/.

become very sick, and guess where they look for help and quick cures? Medications. And what do those medications do? Just like the skin creams and steroids I was given, they put a temporary Band-Aid on a system that is rotting from the inside out. A Band-Aid has no ability to cure you. The great news is that you do! That is why I say, take control of your health, and take control of it from the inside out.

On the Alkaline Sisters blog are two "alkaline vs. acidic" food charts that have helped me immensely, as well as the chart that I have included here by pHreshproducts.com.[15]

pHresh Products acid/alkaline food chart					Learn more at: www.phreshproducts.com	
	highly acidic	moderately acidic	mildly acidic/ neutral	mildly alkaline	moderately alkaline	highly alkaline
Beverages	Alcohol, Soft drinks	Coffee, Black Tea, Processed pasteurized fruit juices	Tap water, Most Bottled water	Coconut Water (without sugar) Natural Spring Water	Green Tea	Lemon Water, Herbal Teas, Alkaline Water, Mineral-Rich Spring Water, Green Juices (juicing greens)
Sweeteners	White Sugar, High Fructose Corn Syrup, Artificial Sweeteners	Processed Honey, Cane Sugar, Brown Sugar	Brown Rice Syrup, Maple Syrup (unprocessed)	Raw Agave Nectar, Raw Honey, Raw Sugar		Raw Stevia (whole leaf)
Fruits		Cranberry, Prune, Most Dried Fruit	Plums, Sour Cherry, Blackberry	Cherry, Orange, Dates, Strawberry, Banana, Peach, Blueberry, Raspberry	Avocado, Fig, Pineapple, Melon, Grape, Kiwi, Raisin, Apple, Pear	Mango, Watermelon, Papaya, Young Coconut, Goji Berry, Citrus Fruit except Oranges and Tomatoes
Vegetables	Commercial Pickles		White Potato	Olives, Button Mushrooms, Tomatoes, Eggplant, Maca Root	Beet, Squash, Zucchini, Cabbage, Carrot, Pepper, Sweet Potato, Cauliflower, Lettuce, Celery, Maitake-Shitake, Reishi Mushroom	Onion, Garlic, Sprouts, Asparagus, Broccoli, Watercress, Ginger, Cucumber, Greens (spinach, kale, leafy greens), Herbs (parsley, cilantro), Sea Vegetables (kelp, spirulina), Grasses (wheat, barley, oat) Fermented Vegetables
Beans/Legumes					All Sprouted Beans	
Grains	Refined Cereal, White & Wheat Flour and Pasta	White Rice, Rye, Corn, Spelt, Unrefined Cereal	Brown Rice, Oat, Buckwheat, Sprouted Whole Grain Bread	Quinoa, Amaranth, Millet, Wild Rice	All Sprouted Grains	
Nuts, Oils, Seeds	Hydrogenated Vegetable Oil, Lard, Refined Oil	Cashews, Walnuts, Peanuts, Pecans	Canola Oil, Safflower Oil (non-refined)	Chestnuts, Almonds, Most Seeds	All Sprouted Nuts & Seeds, Flax Seed / Coconut / Hemp Seed & Olive Oils (Raw / Cold pressed)	
Eggs, Dairy, Non-Dairy	Processed Cheese, Pasteurized Homogenized Cow's Milk products with Added Sugar	Eggs, Pasteurized Homogenized Cow's Milk Products	Pasteurized Goat's Milk Products, Processed Whey, Rice Milk, Raw Cow Milk Products	Almond Milk, Coconut Milk, Raw Whey, Hemp, Raw Goat's Milk (unsweetened)	Breast Milk	
Meats	Conventional Beef, Pork, Shellfish	Grass-fed Beef, Turkey, Chicken, Lamb, Fish	Wild game (venison, ostrich) Cold Water Fish			
Condiments	White Distilled Vinegar, Table Salt (NaCl) Soy Sauce, Commercial Jams, Jelly & Mayonnaise	Ketchup, Mustard	Balsamic Vinegar, Tamari (fermented sauce with sea salt) Homemade Jams, Mayonnaise made with canola oil & sea salt	Mustard made with apple cider vinegar, Most Dried Spices	Apple Cider Vinegar	Himalayan Salt
Eat Less			◀◀◀ ▶▶▶			Eat More

Note: We recommend using organic products whenever possible.

*These statements have not been evaluated by the Food and Drug Administration. Products are not intended to diagnose, treat, prevent or cure any disease.

I stumbled across these wonderful websites while doing my research. I was so appreciative because the charts are easy

15 Alkaline Food Chart, Alkaline Sisters: http://www.alkalinesisters.com/alkaline-food-chart/ and pHreshproducts Charts: http://www.phreshproducts.com/learn/charts/. A special thanks to pHreshproducts.com for allowing me to use this chart with photo credit given to Jeff Stuchala.

to follow and you can carry a copy with you when you shop. Both sites also post alkaline recipes, which are so helpful when you are making this lifestyle change and have to become creative in the kitchen—which I am so *not*! If you ask him, Mike will gladly tell you how many meals I ruined because I wandered off a recipe and got "creative." It's a big joke in our house, and I share a few of these stories later on when I discuss the benefits of actually following a recipe.

Do you remember that old saying, "Eat your veggies?" Well, now your life is not only about eating veggies, but eating *more* veggies and *that* is not an easy task. My problem, in the beginning, was trying to incorporate more veggies into my life on a daily basis. Vegetables are the healers, and they are the one food group I think most people don't get enough of in their diet. I slowly struggled, but now I know my meals are not complete without a veggie. If I am at work and don't have the time to make any or don't have any in my refrigerator, I go out of my way to order some veggie or salad from a nearby restaurant. While this is not my preference, it's nice to know it's an option when you're desperate to get in your greens for the day.

Working in New York City makes it pretty easy to grab some cooked or raw veggies, but when I'm home in Long Island, it's not as easy. You have to go to the store, buy them, come home, prep and cook them. Sometimes there just isn't time to do that. I've learned to have them always on hand, so when I do my big food shop once a week, I buy a ton and fill up my bottom refrigerator drawer. That always gets me through the week. There are the occasional organic veggies that don't make it to day four, but I try hard to use them in some capacity. Usually, I'll juice them, just to avoid wasting them. Also, to be honest with you, there are some days when I just don't want a veggie, period.

One big thing I now do to make sure I always have veggies in the house is I buy them fresh, cut them up, and freeze them. Believe it or not, they taste great if you eat them in the first week or two. I don't like buying frozen veggies because I feel they lose flavor and are a bit too mushy when cooked. But, buying fresh veggies like organic broccoli, cutting them up and freezing them to use within a week or two is different. They still taste awesome! I put the chopped veggies in a Ziploc bag or Tupperware and throw them in the freezer knowing I have plenty for that week in case I run out. I also love to freeze small Ziploc bags of spinach or kale to use in my smoothies! I'll buy a few bags of greens, portion them out, and freeze them to use all week long. I'll get into what I put in my smoothies in a bit, but just know you don't have to rush to use all of your spinach before it goes bad. I always recycle my Ziploc bags, too, so I'm not being wasteful. When I used to work in the city at an office, I would get in my "breakfast veggies" every day by juicing or making a smoothie. I'd have a big glass of kale, celery, romaine lettuce, broccoli, cucumber, apple, lemon, and ginger. It doesn't sound delicious, but *it is*. Maybe I'm just used to it, but I think it's a great sign that my day is not complete without it. I used to wake up early and make the juice first thing in the morning, but sometimes I just couldn't squeeze it in. Some mornings, I started my day at 5:30 a.m. to get to the gym before work. There was no time, and I was not going to sacrifice my workouts to make juice. I found myself making it at night and storing it in airtight mason jar containers (for up to three days). I would fill it all the way to the top to prevent oxidation.

Why did I do that, you ask? Think about when you slice open an apple and it is exposed to the air; it starts turning brown right away. Once you make juice, it gets exposed to the air, and the amount of nutrients will decrease by the day. To prevent this as much as possible, I always include half a lemon in my juices — which helps minimize oxidation — and make sure I fill the jar to the tippy-top, leaving zero room for oxygen.

I've read a number of books on juicing, and most say not to store juice and always to make it fresh because the beneficial nutrients start to dissipate minutes after it's made; you won't be getting all the value consuming the juice days after. But eventually, you just have to admit there's only so much time you have every day. I've also read they can last up to three days: as long as they are in airtight containers, you will get at least some nutrients. I just go with my gut. I also know right away from the taste if the batch is still good. Usually, it still tastes pretty great. I look at it this way: it's better to drink my veggies than not. Nowadays, living with my husband — whom I've turned into a juice hound — the juices don't last longer than a day, anyway! I also always make sure to drink it fresh on the weekends when I have more morning time.

Now that I'm working from home, I'm able to make it fresh more often, which is lovely. Lately, I've been making smoothies a lot since Mike loves to bring them to work. Simple Green Smoothies has a great site with lots of awesome recipes.[16] The secret to their smoothie recipes is the portions. It's basically two cups of leafy greens (typically, spinach or kale), mixed with two cups of water, coconut water, or almond or coconut milk. After mixing that, you throw in two cups of fruit. This makes enough for two smoothies, which is perfect for Mike and me. If you are making it for yourself, cut everything in half. As a word of caution, I would recommend cutting the fruit down to 1/8 cup if you are struggling with anything where you

16   http://www.simplegreensmoothies.com.

should be limiting your sugar intake, such as diabetes, heart disease, candida, obesity, etc. I will get into sugar a bit later, but please know that even though fruit contains natural sugar and is very healthy, it's still sugar, and the yeast that lives in our guts will feed on it and grow and may cause more issues for you. A healthy smoothie means greens with a little flavoring, not a bunch of fruit with a token leaf of spinach! For those of you with a sweet tooth, try to cut down when you can. If the smoothie recipe calls for two cups of fruit, I'm sure 1/8 cup will be sweet enough. If not, you can always add a few drops of Stevia, a teaspoon of organic vanilla, or even better, cut a real vanilla bean and use its seeds. That will give you a lot of flavor. If you are a chocolate nut, add pure cocoa with a little stevia and you will get your fix in no time. If you're finding the cutback too dramatic, try reducing your sugar intake gradually. Your body might not even notice it then. The amazing thing about the healing process is that when you start to cut down on sugars, your sweet-tooth cravings diminish, and you'll find yourself desiring less of the fruit and craving more of the green goodness. How exciting is that?

One of my favorite smoothies—because I am allowed fruit—is using pineapple, mango, or strawberries with banana. So delicious! I used to buy frozen cut up fruit in the store until I discovered it tasted sweeter to me when I bought it fresh, cut it up myself, and froze it. I feel the same way now about kale and spinach. You can buy anything frozen; so if it's easier for you to do that than managing it fresh, I understand. Whatever gets you motivated to drink your greens!

Life has changed for me these last few years, not the least of which because I've managed to make veggies a staple in my everyday diet. My day doesn't feel the same without my veggies, which is a good sign. I love sautéing kale, asparagus, broccoli, okra, spinach—you name it, I find a way to love it. I actually plan my meals around veggies. Mike will ask me what we are doing for dinner, and my answer is usually, "I'm making broccoli and kale." This usually gets me a "That's it?" Of course, there's more, but my thoughts go to what veggies I'm making first. I think this way about lunch as well. I might add brown rice, beans, or tofu to the veggies, but it's all about the veggies!

I understand that it's not easy to always prep and plan, which is what I feel we need to do if we want to heal our skin. It took me a long time to not feel prepping and planning was hard anymore. I go into the details of what to buy and eat in Chapter Seven, and also discuss eating out and its challenges (so, if you need to skip there now, feel free!)

It took me a long time to accept this is the way I would need to live to succeed. In the past, I chose to eat out all the time or ordered in. I relied on other people cooking my food without ever really knowing what was in it. Don't get me wrong; I love taking a break from cooking and enjoy exploring new restaurants, ordering in, or going out once or twice a week. Just remember, though, that taking control of our health means cooking our own food so we know what goes into our bodies.

I would suggest you write down every veggie you know or that you like. Then, go to the store and anything you don't recognize, *try* it. That's the only way you will grow your veggie options. I hear many people say to me they only like broccoli and can't eat it every day. I know for a fact those people have not tried everything in the store. Buy something exotic and ask the internet for a way to cook it. I was very serious about healing my skin, and I had to make serious changes to my diet. The most important change you'll ever make is to increase your veggie intake. I say that from a very loving and experienced part in my heart. Plus, you expand your palate and learn to cook exotic meals.

When I first started this lifestyle, I lived in New York City, and was within a few blocks from a Whole Foods. First of all, is it me or is it not the most beautiful, most colorful store you've ever walked into? The packed displays and shelves of different vegetables are like a rainbow of colors. Though I shop mostly at Trader Joe's to save money, when I needed something specific for my creative chef side, I'd usually find it at Whole Foods. Every time I stepped onto the escalator to go down into that store, I got this giddy, excited feeling in my tummy. I felt like a kid in a candy store when all those colorful fruits and veggies slowly revealed themselves to me as I descended. I'm so cheesy, I know! Food has always had that effect on me. I got that from my dad. Growing up, he loved watching people enjoy eating. We both love everything food-related.

On one specific visit, a man who worked there nicely asked me if I needed help finding anything. While he was helping me, we started to chat about what I was going to bake, which led us into a full-blown inspirational chat about eating alkaline vs. acidic. He told me about this other employee who worked there who eight months prior had been diagnosed with multiple sclerosis. The man was told by his doctor if he didn't go on the recommended prescribed medications he would suffer uncomfortable to extremely painful symptoms. Working at Whole Foods, this guy knew about the healing effects of food and decided to see how using food as his medicine would work. Eight months later, eating mostly alkaline, he hadn't experienced one symptom. I just love that inspirational story.

I have heard so many stories over the years about healing through food; it really doesn't matter what disease we are talking about here. They are all the same in a way. Eating the wrong food causes *dis-ease*, right? I left the store smiling ear to ear because I was beyond inspired and so happy for that person. I knew the universe was pointing me in this direction so clearly. I know I sound very happy eating mostly alkaline, and I'm well aware that's not the norm. Most people would resist it like the plague, but don't forget it took me living with Ps for twenty-one years. I was nineteen years old when I was diagnosed, and I was thirty-five when I had my first complete healing. Experiencing the true effects of this healing is what led me to the ultimate happiness I feel today. I don't think I can ever go back now, and I'm fine with that. I won't lie to you; I have my bad days here and there, but it's rare, and that is honestly more of the tricks that the mind plays on us about wanting what others have or being referred to as "different" versus being happy we have found something to heal our bodies.

I want you to start easy, and before I jump into all things dietary, my next chapter focuses on taking a moment to acknowledge the significance of big transitions in our lives and how to handle them. This, for you, is a big transition, and I just want to give you some good supportive advice to help you through it! But for now, ask yourself: if you knew the difference between alkaline and acidic before—i.e., healthy vs. sick—wouldn't you have already changed your diet? Would you ever leave that basil plant with no water?

While I leave you to ponder the next meditation and prepare for eating right, please remember that from all my research and experience on this diet, I know and want you to know that *no* disease can survive in an alkaline environment. As I said, a Band-Aid has no ability to cure you, but the great news is, you do! That is why I say take control of your health and take control of it from the inside out. If you need a visual to keep you motivated, think of a battery when the acid spills and leaks out and corrodes everything in its track. Now, relate the unhealthy acidic foods to that happening to your body; then, think of the lush green growth of budding spring with all the greens and you will already be on your way to visualizing healing and ultimate health — and here's a side effect you will like, you will be living a psoriasis-free life!

Ps: Let food be *your* medicine.

Meditation

It's time to eat more foods that nourish you. Make a promise to yourself to find these alkaline foods and ways to enjoy them. No more Band-Aids. You are ready to heal and to feel so wonderful in your skin! You've suffered enough. It is time. Feel the empowerment and confidence that comes with taking control of your health. Think about what it feels like to love your skin. It's like nothing else in the world. This will show the universe how much you love yourself, and I promise it will bring you renewed energy, stamina, hope, strength, and so much more. Stay positive and know that I am proud of you for having made it this far and how, even if unconsciously, you are already committing to a change and to a cleansing!

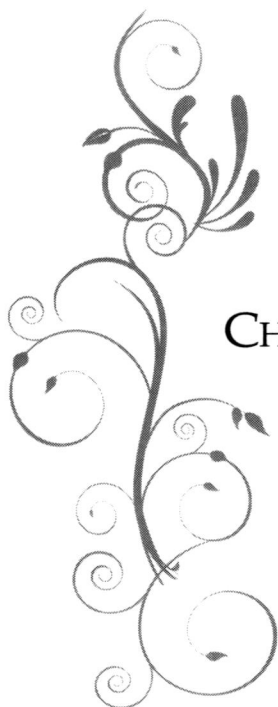

CHAPTER FIVE

Transition

You must be the change you
wish to see in the world.

Mahatma Gandhi

I know that you have just embarked on one of the biggest transitions of your life. Trust me, I know! I've been there. As a matter of fact, I'm in the midst of one now, while writing this book and working so hard to share the message of what I have learned the hard way. My transition is way bigger than I could have ever expected, so I know what you are going through. For me, it was that everything was happening in a short time, so it felt incredibly overwhelming, but in a good way. Within a few months, I had gotten married, turned forty, launched my business, Healing My Skin, and was halfway through writing this book. There were even more exciting life-changing events happening, and the horizon was looking more promising and scarier every moment.

This is most likely what you are experiencing now, as you try to decide if you will trust me enough to take this journey and jump on the alkaline bandwagon. I know that it's hard, I know trusting is hard, and I even know the "deer caught in the headlight" moments and the mind tricks that we play on ourselves and our bodies. Therefore, I just want to share a few emotions I felt going through all this and provide a few suggestions to keep you motivated to make it. Because if you stick to this plan, I guarantee, you will make it!

When we are in the midst of a life-altering event—whether it is a death, an illness, or something positive, a marriage, a birth, a new business, whatever it may be—there are moments that it becomes all surreal, which is truly the best word to describe it. So, the very first piece of advice is that if you keep it positive and if you move with an enlightened goal in mind, you will discover that when you go out of your way to become your best self, really magical things will happen. What I mean by becoming your best self is everything from taking control of your health, to chasing and believing in your dreams, to everything in between.

The in between means taking stock of every moment in your life and working to find more happiness in each one of them. And I use the word *work* because being conscious of our behaviors and our attitudes is a huge part of what leads us to become our best self, but it's not easy. It is not always the things on the outside that make us happy; often, it is the thoughts and beliefs from the inside that need to be modified so that we can make the best of situations around us. Taking mindful and compassionate control of these moments, dousing them with self-love, and then moving forward in our practical day-to-day affairs is what truly defines being our best self—at least in my mind.

Once you nurture your mind, then it is time to work on the external in-betweens, such as taking time to exercise (even if only for twenty minutes), spending more time with friends or family, trying a new veggie with dinner, tackling one little task you might have been putting off (that you know will feel like a burden lifted when complete), or anything that gets you feeling good about trying to move forward—even though some days that might seem impossible.

The point is that when we develop and work on creating our best self, we are doing the most important thing, nourishing ourselves with self-love, and this is key to a happy and healthy life. It could be anything from thinking of two things you are grateful for before going to sleep, to saying "I love you" to yourself in the mirror, to whatever that extra loving thing is that will somehow pass along the beautiful message to the universe that you want *more* of these things in your life because it makes you feel so good. Just remember, you get what you expect, so go ahead and expect things in your life to get better, easier, and happier! Expect your skin to be clear and those spots of psoriasis to fade away. What have you got to lose by expecting the best for your life? In my opinion, you will only gain!

My new transition, as I'm sure will be true of yours, has brought up some terrifying yet exhilarating emotions in me. Luckily, the exhilarating emotions far outweigh the terrifying ones. But, even though wonderful things are happening, there is still stress involved. It is good to remember this when you are going through a stressful time. When I used to audition for parts, I would be so grateful I had the opportunity to act that day. It was wonderful. But along with it came the fear of being judged or not doing well. My nervous system felt unsafe in that room, and I would sometimes find myself shaking. I would plow through it, though, because I refused to let the fear stop me. Even if I came out of there feeling awesome, it was still stress on my body. Keep that in mind, whatever you're doing—starting a new job, going on a date, or a trip, whatever great thing it is—there will always be stress that comes along with it in some way. It's how you handle the stress that matters.

My average day during the stressful times is a game of ping-pong in my brain with thoughts that look like this:

"Move the hell over, fear. You are not standing in my way!"

"Can I do this? Okay, breathe, Kim!"

"Hell, yeah, I got this!"

"What if I'm not good enough and fail?"

"I always believed I was supposed to do something big. This is it!"

I can assure you: you are not the only person whose mind can race all day long!

Somewhere in my body, I'm scared and shaking. But, at the same time, I've *never* felt so happy and ecstatic. I've been walking around super-overwhelmed, yet on cloud nine! Have you ever felt both yin and yang at the same time? It's stressful on our bodies, and I realize I need to calm the hell down. I know that all those ping-pong thoughts are not good for anyone.

Because I am just like everyone else (human!) I want to share my four go-to tricks that work best for me to get myself grounded and quiet my racing thoughts so that I'm not all over the place. Perhaps when you are feeling a bit yin and yang, these will help you as well:

1. Step outside, ground your feet (especially if there is some place you can take your shoes off and step on the grass), take a walk—even if it's just around the block.

2. Meditate, even if it is only for two minutes, and even if it is just taking a succession of deep breaths in and out, five seconds for each, a few times in a row.

3. Step away from the electronics, silence your phone for one minute, turn off all the external computer, TV, music, and auxiliary noise and listen to the beauty of silence.

4. And, my ultimate favorite, watch the synchronicity of the birds flying above. You can do this while you are walking around the block. You can walk to your window and look up. For this, I'd even let you look at this on a computer screen, because looking at the synchronicity of the birds is like looking at fish swimming in a fish bowl; it calms the mind and can physically reduce your heart rate. I always watch the birds while I'm waiting for the train. I can't help but seek them out, up there on that platform.

Strange, but now birds find me! Or maybe they've been here the whole time, and I'm just finding them now. I'll be driving and, out of nowhere, a huge flock of them will gracefully fly by in such incredible unity. It is amazing. It forces me into the present moment more than anything else. The moon does that for me as well. I *love* to stare at the moon. You get my point. Find anything in nature, in its perfect creation, to focus on, and you will find your mind has taken a quick break from its worries. When is the last time you stopped working or talking on the phone to admire a beautiful tree or flower?

It's time. Your transition time is here, so think about the exciting things you are on the verge of. Think of how you are going to be healed soon. Think about how you are going to be the person who will give yourself self-love at all times, and think about having your mind and body merge in the unified and beautifully loving way that you deserve. Know that you are loved. Actively work to do things that will make you happier. Try out a few of my suggestions and know that your body was designed to heal. The way the universe sends the flock of birds to your life, the way they work in unison — that is what your body can and will do for you. So, transition for the better. Stay hopeful and know that if you need help, motivation, a shoulder to cry on, or a word of encouragement, I am here for you.

Remember, you get what you expect. I always expect to have an impact on this world, and so should you. What would happen if we all expected greatness and moved the universe in that direction? Greatness would be achieved. Now *that* gives me chills. And that is what motivates me to want to help you make the transition. Hold on! We are about to embark on the biggest moment and change in your life, and I'm here for you.

☜

Ps: Like the caterpillar, you are about to spin your cocoon and rise to a new level of love and health, and for this, I salute you.

Meditation

Think positive and don't allow negative thoughts in your transition. A negative thought will enter the mind and, before you know it, another one and another one. Pay attention, visualize those thoughts being blown out of a window, then shut the window and replace them with positive thoughts. Tell yourself, "I will make a concerted effort not to allow negative thoughts to overcome me, and if one enters my mind, I will consciously replace it with a positive thought, because I embody love and I manifest healing." And now, from this point on, no matter what you see, what you hear, or what you feel, you tell yourself over and over, "I have already transitioned. It is done. I am healed." Because, my dear friend, you are.

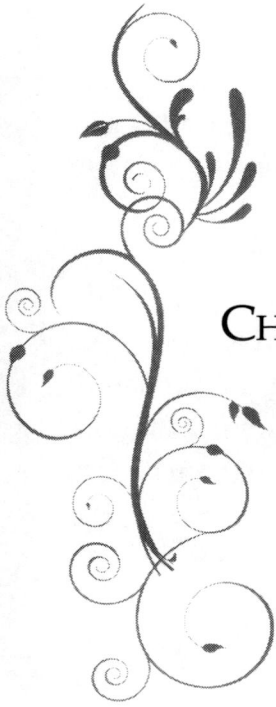

CHAPTER SIX

Learning Unconditional Acceptance

*The secret to change is to
focus all of your energy,
not on fighting the old,
but on building the new.*

Socrates

One of the most valuable lessons that I have learned to date is that change is never easy. Whether it is a change in relationships, a change in style, a change in behavior, a change in health—no matter the situation, we all face even a small bit of change with trepidation. As I mentioned in Chapter Five, the change relating to my life transitions was a happy one, yet stressful. For you, it could be an anxiously awaited and joyful change, like having a baby, starting a business, taking a trip to unknown lands. For others, it may an unwanted change due to a long illness, death, divorce, or a move. For some strange reason, the one common denominator in humans is that, whether sad or happy, people are resistant to change.

For this reason, I want to share what it takes to be successful in behavior modification, and in our case, the change for the *better* because this is what this book is all about. The secret, as Socrates says, is "to focus all of your energy, not on fighting the old, but on building the new."

Why is it that for hundreds of years, and our entire lifetimes, we still resist this one easy secret to success? I recently experienced an emotional episode in my life that is the perfect example of resistance to change, and now that it has passed, and I have integrated it, I feel compelled to share it with you. I must admit, this was originally not going to be in this book, but the more I thought about the process and its impact, the more I felt it was crucial for you to have this valuable piece of information.

I will begin by saying that I don't want ever to pretend that life is always perfect for me. Just like you, a part of any person's healing process is the acceptance of change. Again, having been described as that positive and patient person with a constant smile on my face and slow to anger, life isn't any more perfect for me than for you. I am sharing this life episode with you to offer encouragement and support, and quite frankly to share together, so that we can all heal more quickly.

As of the last few years, I have learned to make it a point to show others what is in my heart because I feel that by sharing my personal struggles I can teach others what a healing process looks like. This way when you have a crisis, you will be able to try these behavior modification steps for yourselves, especially since, some days, no one can pull you through your own crap but you!

This story is about body image. For as long as I can remember, I've been hiding my body. I love my parents to death, but I don't love the genetic makeup I've inherited. We are a family with wide curvy hips and slender legs that, on me, seem to gain weight only at the tippy-top of the thigh area. Now, I know, small petite women out there may be very envious of my womanly curves, and everyone knows "we all want what we don't got," right?

As a child, I was always naturally thin, skinny actually. While writing this, I'm sitting here looking at my dance re-cital photo from when I was probably around ten, and, boy, was I a skinny-minnie! I'm not saying that I want that body back, and having recently turned forty, I'm not even upset at aging; but, I can say that deep within my mind there are still little demons that pop-up now and then to remind me they can control my thoughts, shock me out of blissfulness, and immediately destroy my self-esteem.

Allow me to describe what I mean. Growing up, I learned about negative body image and the constant need to do bet-ter, look better, be better. Probably like many of you, it was partially by watching my mom and seeing her pursue endless diets. She was the classic yo-yo dieter. She was on Weight Watchers on-and-off my entire life—so much so that it be-came normal. Even then, everything on TV and everything about growing up seemed to circle back to how we look and the need to compare ourselves to others. In case you haven't realized, the movie and advertising industries were not cre-ated to make being the norm good enough. Let's face it, few of us look like Julia Roberts or Jennifer Garner.

I truly don't remember when I started to worry about my looks and to yo-yo diet myself, but I'm sure it was sometime during college, when I was messing around with boys and feeling that typical insecurity young girls feel. As our hor-mones change and our bodies grow, and as we age, we all ex-perience changing physiques. It's nature. What is not natural is being ashamed and embarrassed by it. Animals don't hang around saying, "Wow, I have a couple of gray whiskers that weren't there a few years ago and, man, look at that pouch I'm now sporting!" I doubt women in reclusive Amazonian tribes hang out discussing how rough their feet have gotten from walking in the jungle barefoot or how saggy their boobs have become after twelve children. This is because of the one simple mental trick that has been played on us through the years: they have not been inundated their whole lives by an entertainment industry telling them what pretty is or is not. No one is forcing them to live up to those advertising images on TV and in magazines and telling them what's fashionable or not, or what body shape is ideal.

That's just it, isn't it? The pressure of what others tell us is the norm, and us giving these messages credence — *believing* them — is what actually creates the self-consciousness about our bodies. If we refused the false advertising, if we never put conditions on our beauty, then that little mind devil could never pop up to torture us. We would not buy into feeling unworthy or ugly if we don't look like the Victoria Secret model or an A-list actress on the red carpet. We wouldn't tell ourselves, "If we aren't Barbie, we'll never get married." We would never believe there is something wrong or inadequate or horrible about ourselves, and our bodies, and as a result, become self-conscious, critical, and not exercise our right to unconditional acceptance.

Unconditional acceptance! That is what this chapter is about.

Until that one special incident that made me write about this, I had never really focused on the specifics of when this mind-game of falling for a false or impossible attainment of body composition first happened to me. All I know is that, from a young teen until even now in my forties, I have felt self-conscious about my body. I remember, during my college years, going out in the dead of winter in clothing that did nothing to keep me warm! In those days, fashion always trumped reason. I must have had some confidence about my body to wear what I wore back then. So, I ask myself, when did this deep-rooted feeling of not being enough start and, even worse, why did it just re-reveal itself in this recent episode?

Here's when and why my little meltdown happened. I had come off a high of so many wonderful, yet stressful, things happening at one time. It all came to a head after I returned home from an awesome shopping experience with a dear friend. I was in Los Angeles and, for a few hours, I *was* Julia Roberts in *Pretty Woman*. My fashion guru friend and I had an exceptional time, during which she felt comfortable enough (and that is not always easy) to point out that I don't wear things that flatter my beautiful shape enough. She is not the only one that has pointed this out (and my husband would be thrilled if I dressed a little sexier). I left there from a whirlwind shopping spree with clothes galore for my new profession and was thrilled with the time and the experience. It was such a gift, and to this day I'm so grateful to her for the love she showed me.

What I didn't realize, until a few days later, was how much "hiding" my body and the positive feedback that "I should" feel comfortable wearing more form-fitting clothes was eating away at me. I mean, I know that I tend to hide my curves in my hippy, dippy, flowy clothes, but I freaking love that style!

When I returned home, I found myself shopping last minute in Anthropologie because I had a gift card and needed an engagement dress. Everything in that store is so me, very hippie and flowy. I wanted to buy everything, but after texting images of several choices to friends, I could tell no one was happy, and they were gently trying to say my choices were not flattering enough to my body. This was when the meltdown happened, and when the voices in my head started having it out:

Devil: "Don't buy that, it doesn't flatter you."

Angel: "Embrace your shape and own it."

Devil: "That's not fitted enough."

Angel: "Loose is fine. You are beautiful. You can wear anything."

Then, *I* got involved: "But I like these hippie clothes," I said to the devil, along with a long list of other statements, like, "I should have bought clothes that had more color when I was in Los Angeles. Why do I have to change? What's wrong with the way I am? What's wrong with me?"

While shopping and texting, I couldn't help but think, "Where were all these questions coming from and why was I soon to be an emotional sobbing wreck because of them?" When I dug deep, I realized what the answer was, and I didn't like it: I want to make *others* happy, and I want them to *approve* of me. That's where the battle was. The battle wasn't figuring out want I wanted — I wanted to buy all those flowy dresses. In my mind, they didn't want me to be *me,* and they wouldn't approve. However, another part of me also wanted so badly to want to *not* cover up; I wanted to *want* the tighter clothes!

The pressure between wanting to please them and wanting to remain comfortable as to who I had become (most likely because of the Ps and the endless barrage of "ideal" body types) was rearing its ugly head. These people love me. I know this. They want the best for me. So why was I so very hurt?

And then the "aha" moment occurred, and I was pulled back to images of when I was nineteen. I began to wonder if this is why my psoriasis manifested, to give me more of what I was putting out there, more to hide from the world? I was hiding my family life. I was putting a smile on my face to make others happy, and I was already covering up the Ps by nineteen; and from that point on, it became second nature to spend my life covering up. That's what I knew; therefore, that is who I became.

A few days later and after much analysis, I asked myself, when am I going to accept and approve of myself enough to let down that veil of shame and to embrace my body for all its imperfections and perfections? Had I created a safety zone in the loose and flowy clothes because I had convinced myself I needed cover, or was this really my look and style?

It saddens me, now, when I think about it because I've wasted so much of this precious life feeling like "not enough" when it's simply not true! I am enough. *We* are enough. You are enough. You are beautiful. And inside you know it. I know it. We know it. We are life and life is beautiful. When are we going to stop beating ourselves up and just focus on loving the crap out of ourselves?

I'm sure every person on the planet can relate to this story and these feelings in some aspect. Some of us want to be perfect, some of us want to be everything to everyone. But why? I now know that we don't want to feel hurt, criticized, or rejected. It took me forty years to figure this out, and that's all it comes down to: loving myself more than ever and accepting the fact that life may hurt or reject me, but that if I practice unconditional *acceptance* with myself, I can live a joyful and healed life.

That is the point you need to determine for yourself: why have you chosen a certain path? A certain style? A certain attitude? But be honest about it. And when you come to terms with it, make the changes until the real *you*, the real *fit* of who you are and want to be emerges. When that time comes, you simply won't give a crap what others think, and you will emerge every time as the real you for the world to love. If others can't accept you that way, well, that is their problem. Stop hiding.

I confess, it is *hard* to have positive and unconditionally loving and accepting thoughts when you are seeing spots of Ps appear, especially while you are eating clean six days a week. Those spots "surfacing" tell me a very different story, an emotional story. I talk a lot more about this in Chapter Nine on emotions, but for this topic, it always takes me back a bit, because my fear comes rushing in and I'm back in that *not enough* head space so quickly, I don't know what hit me. Imagine, here I am writing a book, helping people every day, being this loving, positive light for people and helping them heal, and out of nowhere the little girl in me who feels so helpless pops right in.

The difference, now, is that I know I have the control to heal myself, and I know, in times like these, I need to love the crap out of myself. I know that's the answer, and that's what I want to share with you. In moments like the one at Anthropologie or when we can finally realize we have been acting on a defense mechanism, I don't want you to forget that the mind, body, and spirit are all connected and that we must be our *true* self and not the self others want us to be. That is the only way we will ever be happy. We have to look deeper at what the circumstances are around ourselves, what we are manifesting by our actions, our attitudes, our self-talk, our behaviors, and even by those we surround ourselves with. We have to take note and be willing to make a change. It doesn't mean throwing the baby out with the bathwater. It means consciously working on one small step at a time. Even one small change, as simple as changing a negative thought and rephrasing it to a positive, will change your psyche and then your physical being. It's really an amazing thing we can do if we just try even a little bit!

I want you to think for a moment about a simple yawn. Everyone has experienced watching someone yawning and then suddenly needing to as well. It's contagious and automatic. Now, think of a smile and a laugh. Do you know the beauty in the fact that if someone smiles and laughs there is a good chance you will too? Now, think of a moody, brooding individual who is always negative. That will bring your energy down in seconds. So choose to walk away from those negatives and move on to the people or things that make you smile, shine, or laugh!

I know deep in my heart the message I'm meant to share with the world is about unconditional acceptance. We must learn to do and think about everything from this new perspective. It feels so hard sometimes, which I'm learning on my journey, but that's the contrast I need to experience to learn this lesson of unconditional acceptance. Sometimes the scaffolding we are building our lives on will feel like it has come crashing down and we are left feeling helpless and confused.

Instead of falling with it, try to confront the things so that fear does not hold you back.

Franklin D. Roosevelt said, "There is nothing to fear but fear itself," and I could not agree more. A friend reminded me, in my time of fear, that I was not alone, that many people out there are always feeling it too, even in that exact moment you are. I can't explain why, but this made me feel better. It always feels better not to be alone, especially during dark times. Fear has a way of bringing what should be excitement in certain situations to a screeching halt. It can make us lose our breath and make our hearts feel like they are going to beat out of our chest. Fear is not a terrible thing; it was created to protect us from danger. It enables our body to go into "fight or flight" mode when something is threatening our survival. The fear I'm referring to pops into our heads on a daily basis from simply not feeling good enough. This fear can be devastating if you allow it to be. It can sabotage that promotion, the hot date, good news—and worst of all, your self-worth! Don't allow that fear to stop you from doing what you were put on this earth to do, which is to find happiness and joy and to share love every day.

When fear pops up, please remember it's the universe's little reminder that you *should* face it, whatever *it* is, that it *is* worth it. I can't tell you how many articles and books I have read where people say you should do something that scares you every day. I think that's a little too scary for a lot of people, so they hold back and play it safe. In those moments, ask yourself, who is telling you to be afraid? No one can make you feel fear, only you. Next time you feel it, just breathe your way through it and accept where you're at, at that moment. Remind yourself that you *are* good enough. This is where that switch from negative thoughts to positive thoughts becomes *key*! Face it, analyze it, talk to it. I'm not saying this will make the fear go away forever, but what it will do is break that vicious cycle and help you move toward what scares you so you can release it. When you move toward it, you will conquer it little by little noticing the next time won't feel so hard. You will move toward unconditionally accepting all the parts of yourself.

And, as per my body image breakdown and story, although this particular day was more than painful and it had me shaking and sobbing and trying to find my breath, I realized that whatever I needed to release was pretty powerful. I want to help you learn that on those days, breathe into the fear, into the feelings. Let go of feeling like you're not enough, but don't avoid or repress the thoughts, because if we do, they will negatively manifest in some other way, shape, or form. Feeling our feelings is one of the hardest things, but we must, for positive change and healing to occur.

In a recent talk, Kris Carr said that, even after becoming a *New York Times* bestselling author and helping thousands of people, she found herself feeling broken about the fact that she still has cancer in her body. On one particular day, she was walking in the woods feeling down about this when a bee literally came from the sky, hit her right on her third eye, and fell to its death. She giggled telling the story, and it *was* quite funny. This bee came from the universe with a strong message for her that she got right away: she *can* have a long, rich, healthy life *with* cancer. She said it was all about unconditional acceptance, not giving up, and never abandoning yourself. It's about owning your self-worth, respecting yourself, honoring who you are at *this* moment, not when you get to where you want to be.

We all want to feel better and be better, but we create more suffering in our lives when we live from a place of not enough. She pointed out that none of us are broken, we don't need fixing—we just need loving. I heard this and thought, *What a relief; we are enough!* I took a deep breath and realized my little meltdown was my message from the universe, which was to love, accept, and approve of myself *with* or *without* Ps, with or without weight, imperfections, and all those other body image issues.

These experiences come to tell us there is something off-balance in our lives. We need to appreciate them and love the messenger. We must choose love, and we must choose to love our body enough never to abandon it again. It is a process, and we can't do it all overnight, but we can take one more step. We can do that with simple thoughts like *I am enough. I have a beautiful body. I am healed. I am comfortable in this skin. I love my body. My body is good to me!*

Remember, our beliefs are just thoughts we keep thinking over and over again; that's all they are. They are thoughts and we have the option to keep them as-is, where they can negatively impact us, or we can choose to modify them into positive thoughts. Let's work together on making them positive.

One of the beautiful parts about being human is that not one of us is perfect, and not one of us is the same. You all have a story to tell about the days you've abandoned yourself. I hope this encourages you to share your story with others, with me, with us here as a supportive community. Find those who exude and give love and spend less time with those who don't. Teach yourself to forgive and love yourself with all your imperfections even if this is not what you were taught growing up.

Life is a journey. Change is hard. We must embrace building the new self and rid ourselves of the restrictions we placed around ourselves while holding on to the old self.

At the end of the day, I hope this story resonates deep enough that you, too, can extend a hand of *unconditional acceptance* to yourself, as I eventually managed to do that day!

☙

Ps: I love you, now go and love yourself.

Meditation

Today I want you to take a moment, to take this mental test:

Choose one limited belief you have that doesn't serve you. One that hurts the most or you fear the most. Thank it for being your biggest indicator of what change needs to happen in you. Think about how your life would be without this belief. Visualize it. Be conscious during the day when a negative thought enters your mind. Change it to a positive and move on with your day until you have a moment like this meditation to work on where it is coming from. Know that, by releasing the negative somewhere deep in you, it is causing an ever so subtle shift to a happier life. Continue to catch these negative thoughts and change them. By doing so, you will change.

Then, thank the universe for bringing the negative thought to you because, without it, you would never know how delicious your life could be once you make this transition. Thank it one more time before saying goodbye. It served you for a time, but now you're ready to move on to better things. (For example: Thank you Ps for showing me how to eat healthy, love myself, and serve others. You've done a lot for me, and I appreciate you very much. I'll always be grateful you brought me closer to myself and to a more joyful life. I love you, but now it is time to say goodbye.)

What is it that is old that you can give up on so that you can see yourself anew? I don't need fixing, I need loving, and I am now going to go and give that unconditional acceptance to myself!

I want to share one last piece: In a moment of pain, a dear and wise friend wrote me this letter that I would like to share with you:

Insert your name and know you are loved …

Dear _____:

You are a wonderful, incredible, loving, trying so hard to be perfect, being.

The best news is that when the universe steps in and slaps us in the face with a difficult and emotional experience; it is because we are on our way to a breakthrough of mass proportions. The universe does not want us to miss the point again. It wants us to make a change for the better.

It also steps in as a test and sends us a load of negativity to see if we mean what we say and if we believe in our path, our true destiny. This is a sign that you are on the right track. This breakout and breakdown will come and go, and you will see healing again. This is an exercise in belief (some call it faith), but it is proof that you are releasing the old and bringing in a new and more evolved you. You have *not* done something wrong, so do not pick on yourself, do not attack yourself; now is the time to love yourself enough to move into a more enlightened and loving place.

Stay strong, write about it, vent about it, make as much sense of it as you can—but then release it. Like your "condition," thank it for visiting and then allow it to go so that you can get on with your vibrant life because your exciting new path awaits you.

Sending love, Love, LOVE because this will pass, you *will* become stronger, and you *will* learn that the universe just cleared the way for your success.

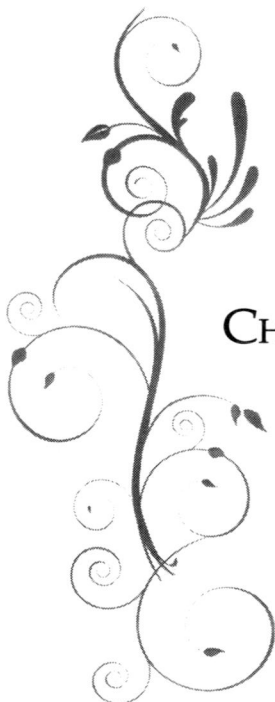

CHAPTER SEVEN

You're Cleaner When You Eat Greener

In a world where dietary choices are poor, environmental pollution is heavy, stress levels are high and exercise is often a last priority, internal cleansing is more important than ever for optimal health.

Dr. Bernard Jensen

The day has begun. You have done your research, set your goals and path, and have decided to dive in and try to clean up your eating act. This chapter is about the practical steps I took as I first learned about the process of turning my body from acidic to alkaline. I am not asking you to necessarily do all of them at once; I am hoping that some of these steps will give you encouragement and the strength to say, "I can do this too!" I also want to help save you from some moments of over-achievement where you think more is better. I promise you it's not, and I will share some funny stories to prove it.

When I first started this journey, five years ago, I was living and working in New York City. I had to be in the office at 10:00 a.m., so I would wake up at 6:00 a.m. and start with a mug of hot water with freshly squeezed lemon. This routine is still the main start to my day. Without it, I just don't feel the same, and I encourage you to do this one thing the rest of your life. New studies are continuously coming out that this one small step can change the acidic level in your body to alkaline, which lasts all day long, and is where you want to be for true health. It is hard to believe that a lemon or lime, which people think of as acidic, can actually make your body alkaline, but trust me, it does.[17] Nearly every nutritionist and naturopath agree that this one step keeps all systems moving and helps you start your day balanced.

While sipping the lemon water, I would get dressed and, by the time I was done, I was ready to start my green juice as my first breakfast. It would be anything from kale, spinach, cucumber, celery, parsley, lemon, apple or ginger to carrots, celery, sweet potato, pineapple, lime, or beets.

Today, my favorite juice of all time, which I make more than any other juice, consists of the following:

- 6 kale leaves
- ½ cucumber
- 4 celery sticks
- Small handful of parsley or mint herbs
- ½ lemon (without the rind)
- 2 golden delicious or gala apples (I use organic apples, so I throw them in whole without removing the seeds and stem.)
- ½ inch of fresh ginger

---

17   If you are a technical person and want to read more information on how this process works, please go to http://www.healthyfoodhouse.com/why-is-lemon-water-alkaline/.

My second favorite is:

- ½ lemon
- 1 sweet potato
- Handful of carrots (I do not juice the fronds.)
- 2 small gala apples
- ½ inch of ginger (I don't take off the outer layer of skin.)

Back then, by the time I got to the office, I would get hungry and need something with more substance. This was when I would have my second breakfast. My go-tos tended to be Ezekiel sprouted bread with almond butter and banana, a piece of fruit with nuts, or oats with almond butter, blueberries, raspberries, or banana and a sprinkle of cinnamon.

I want to take a minute and talk more about Ezekiel bread because it is one of the life-saving food staples I keep on hand, and it is so very good. Like you, I always knew that regular packaged bread from the supermarket was processed so that it could sit on the shelf for weeks without molding. Who doesn't love that squishy, white Wonder bread of the old days? Remember Twinkies? They could last on a shelf for over twenty years! My teacher at the Institute for Integrative Nutrition refers to such things as chemical concoctions. Don't get me started on all the preservatives, artificial colorings, sweeteners, and sugars that go into them. When something is processed, just think of it as being stripped of most of its nutrients. Think of it as putting complete junk food in your body that can rapidly increase aging and illness versus food that can create health and vibrancy.

Sprouted grain bread is a healthy alternative to any unsprouted flour bread because it is made using whole grains that have been soaked in water until they sprout, and only then are the grains ground into flour. This process of soaking and sprouting destroys the phytic acid which can prevent the body from being able to absorb the vitamins and nutrients it needs.[18] I always try to soak brown rice the night before I cook it for this same reason. The nutrients from the grain are then absorbed immediately into our bodies, which is quite the opposite from regular flour bread, whether white or whole wheat. Preserved and processed food is so much harder to digest, and you lose a good amount of nutrients because the body can't fully digest them. It is essential to start learning what foods nourish you versus what foods deplete you.

The health benefits of sprouted grains far outweigh those of white flour or whole wheat flour, and many people don't realize that wheat flour itself is just made up of refined white flour. People don't know this because major companies don't want you to learn what really happens before the food we eat arrives at the grocery store. White flour is made from heavily refined and processed wheat grains. (Key words here: heavily processed.) That usually means it has been stripped of all its nutrients—fiber being a huge one—and most of the vitamins and minerals our bodies need. Ever see the words *fortified* or *enriched* on your bread packages? This means things are *added back* into the bread after being removed during processing. If there is no nutritional benefit left after the grains are so heavily processed that we have to put vitamins and minerals back in, doesn't this alone set off an alarm?

I find it fascinating that science can even do this, and even more fascinating that someone realized our food had no nutrients and pressured some unnamed governing body to put vitamins and minerals back in. It is important to realize,

---

18   http://www.foodforlife.com/about_us/sprouted-grain-difference.

however, that when those vitamins and minerals are added back, they are most likely not even absorbed by our bodies. Even though 100 percent whole wheat flour is better for you because it's made from grains that aren't processed as heavily (so the nutritional value is higher), it still does not provide real nutrition for our bodies.

One thing all this researching and trial and error has taught me is that you have to be an investigator when you go food shopping, and you must learn to inspect the labels. Even though 100 percent whole wheat bread is made using whole wheat flour, you'll see that the ones labeled "whole wheat" may contain both whole wheat and white flours. Some even have caramel coloring added to them to turn the color of the flour brown! Who thought this up? So, be sure the very first ingredient on the label is whole grain or whole wheat. Nothing should be listed first except that, and if it's not, put that chemical concoction back on the shelf and keep looking, or buy sprouted because your body and your skin will thank you later.

Sprouted bread has numerous benefits. It helps us digest and absorb our minerals more easily, provides us with amino acids, extra antioxidants, and has vitamins B and C. It gives our bodies what they need from grains: nutrients. You should know it does naturally contain gluten, like other bread, but they now sell gluten-free brands. A lot of people with skin conditions may have an intolerance to gluten, so in that case, be cautious. If you have no issues with gluten, I urge you to switch it up and see how you feel. If you are craving toast or a sandwich, this can now be your go-to bread. I mean, think about how much bread we eat on a daily basis. Switching to sprouted grains will help you get more of the nutrients you need to heal that skin of yours. Our goal is to indulge in anything that is easier on our digestive tract!

Various companies now make sprouted grain bread, but my favorite is a brand called Ezekiel, which is made by Food for Life. There is no flour in it, only six different sprouted grains. Because there are no preservatives added, I keep it in my freezer at all times. If I want to have a few slices, I'll take out only what I need. My favorite breakfast these days, since I'm now mostly working from home, is two slices of their cinnamon raisin flavored bread, toasted, with a smear of almond butter and some warm gooey strawberry or blueberry sauce. I make the sauce by throwing the berries and a dash of coconut oil in a pot to cook until it boils down. Honestly, you can just throw some cut-up berries on it if you're feeling lazy. Sometimes for lunch, I love having it toasted with hummus and avocado. Both options are so easy and so delicious. You can find this sprouted bread at most health food stores, as well as Whole Foods and Trader Joe's. Once in a while, I'll be surprised and see it in the freezer section of a regular supermarket or even at Walmart.

Now, what if you don't live in an area where you have access to health food stores or even organic food? I must say I was quite spoiled living in New York City for eleven years. Now that I'm out in the suburbs, I miss the convenience and variety that was at my fingertips. There's not the same variety of restaurants, food stores, or cafés on every other corner where I can grab a few healthy items from the salad bar. I am, however, very lucky to have a Trader Joe's and an organic supermarket not too far from my apartment. I also recently discovered a small health food store in my area that I never realized had so much to offer, so I do feel very fortunate. I'm well aware that a lot of towns and cities around the world don't have a health food store that can offer some of the replacement foods I mention in this book or even some of the organic options. Maybe those places are too far away from you, or maybe your budget doesn't allow you to buy healthier foods because they are more expensive. I wish fruits and veggies were subsidized the way corn is in this country. How a bag of carrots or apples is more expensive than a bag of Doritos is beyond me and material for an entirely different book.

I recently spoke to a pen pal I met from chatting on the National Psoriasis Foundation forum about how she eats a lot of red meat. She and her husband really enjoy it, but she's unable to buy grass-fed organic beef because she lives in a small town where that's just not an option. She has to drive two hours to the closest bigger city if she wants to buy it. I suggested she plan a day trip with her husband, explore the sights somewhere near that city, equip themselves with a cooler in the car, and on the way home stop and purchase a bunch of steaks to bring back to freeze. I know this may sound like a pain, but they would enjoy a fun day with whatever adventure they had planned, and it really wouldn't be too much of an inconvenience. I would love doing something like that. I would rather her do that once every few months than continue to eat red meat that is pumped with hormones and antibiotics and sold in your local grocery store.

One suggestion I would make for those of you who are on a tight budget and may want to buy organic, but it's a bit too hard on your wallet, is only to buy organic fruits and veggies on the following list to avoid those that contain the highest amount of pesticides. This list is from the Environmental Working Group, who specialize in research on toxic chemicals and other issues that impact our food, health, and the environment. These are called the Dirty Dozen because they are the most contaminated so you should buy organic whenever possible:[19]

The Dirty Dozen

- Apples
- Celery
- Tomatoes
- Cucumbers
- Grapes
- Nectarines
- Peaches

- Potatoes
- Spinach
- Strawberries
- Blueberries
- Sweet bell peppers
- (Green beans and kale are moving up on the most sprayed list, so beware.)

The Clean Fifteen is another list of fruits and vegetables this group put together.[20] These are the ones that aren't sprayed as heavily and that you can buy non-organic. This gives you peace of mind and saves you money:

The Clean Fifteen

- Onions
- Avocado
- Sweet corn
- Pineapple
- Mango
- Sweet peas
- Eggplant
- Cauliflower

- Asparagus
- Kiwi
- Cabbage
- Watermelon
- Grapefruit
- Sweet potatoes
- Honeydew melon

19   https://www.ewg.org/foodnews/dirty_dozen_list.php.
20   https://www.ewg.org/foodnews/clean_fifteen_list.php.

When you begin to restock your kitchen with healthier alternatives and staples, a great suggestion for those of you who simply don't have the access to a health food store in your area is to shop online. I order everything from chia seeds to coconut oil to herbal tea from Amazon. It's quite amazing when you think about it. If you are a regular shopper like me, you can buy a Prime membership for under $150 for the entire year, and they guarantee you free two-day shipping. Yes, you can receive an order in two days. You can order just about anything online now. I've ordered dried fruit, granola, smoothies, juices, raw snacks—you name it, I've ordered it from various companies all over the world. I recently ordered herbs from India and oils from England. The internet is amazing and can be so helpful with finding resources.

Also, don't forget to ask around in your local shops. Maybe there is a farmer's market by you that visits every other Saturday that you don't even know about. Maybe if enough people ask for these resources, they will start to develop in more areas. Maybe *you* will be the catalyst to that happening. Who knows! Just do the best you can; that's good enough. You don't have to go crazy running around. You have to do what makes you happy, because if finding an organic chicken causes you stress, there's no point in eating it. The last thing I want is for you to have any negative feelings about the food you're consuming. Let food become your friend, respect it, and show it love. I guarantee it'll show you love back. Figure out a few small things you can do that will make a difference in your life and for your skin. Do what makes you feel good, not what makes you feel overwhelmed or completely inconvenienced.

Now that I live in the suburbs, I try to make it a point to stop at my favorite health food store in the city when I pop in to see friends. Just recently, I had a dentist appointment in midtown and was meeting a friend after for lunch. I scheduled the lunch with enough time in between so I could pick up some of my favorite healthy snacks. I stocked up because I knew it would be a while before I got the chance to go there again. Like I said, just do your best and know that is enough. I urge you to hang on because times are changing and lots of people out there are making a difference in our food system. Once you start your journey and are on the lookout for more accessible, nutritious foods, you will slowly start to find ways to get them.

There are even small communities that have started communal gardening. It's such a great venture. You can choose to volunteer and get free veggies in season delivered to your home, or you can pay $140 per person, pre-season, in some states, and get veggies delivered all summer long. It may sound like a lot, but how much do you (or should you) spend on veggies in a three-month period? On top of that, there is nothing better than the flavor of a veggie that was just pulled out of the ground that morning. That, of course, is a ground that is not contaminated.

With the topic of contamination, I am going to digress for a moment before I move on to the lunch menu to discuss the topic of GMOs because it is imperative that you start to pay attention to this when you shop.

My entire life, I never knew that I was eating genetically modified foods (GMOs). Today, I wonder if that had something to do with me developing psoriasis at nineteen. Nutrient-packed food comes from the earth, not laboratories.

Unfortunately, I didn't give this much thought until I was well into my thirties. I knew when I was young that to lose weight I had to eat more fruits and veggies, but that's all I knew. I never stopped eating a bag of Doritos to think, "I have no idea what these ingredients are!" Unfortunately, I don't think many people pay attention to this, still.

I had the most inspiring teacher in class one week who is known as the Food Babe. Yes, the Food Babe! She's an incredible food activist that has a very moving story about taking her health into her own hands. Let's just say that investigating her food saved her life. Since then, she's taken on many of the big food giants and won. She's currently fighting the good fight of trying to get our country to label GMOs (over fifty other countries already require this). How can America boast that we are the richest and best nation in the world, and yet we are feeding our people some of the least-healthy food? We blindly eat and drink these ingredients every day without knowing or being given a choice to do otherwise. This makes me so angry, and I jumped on the Food Babe's bandwagon right away. (Check out her story on her awesome blog, foodbabe.com. You just might become a Food Babe groupie as well.)

Until I started doing my own research, I never knew that GMO foods are injected with new DNA, viruses, herbicides, and chemicals to repel insects *and* resist natural herbicides, and most importantly, to look so perfectly rounded and colorful so that everything looks pretty in the grocery store. Not healthy, mind you, but pretty. I don't want people eating anything that makes them sick and there's just no way that foods injected with anything unnatural can make us well. That leads me to ask: why would the people who run this country allow GMOs at all? There are many studies linking GMOs to over twenty different diseases and this pattern of eating GMOs, getting sick, going to the doctor, taking medication, and in turn, getting more sick is unsustainable! Well, for anyone other than the pharmaceutical companies, GMO-pitching companies, and certain financial organizations.

There has to be a better way to feed our country. The Food Babe says that to be an activist all you need to do is share your story and allow it to affect others, because it will. I guess whether people realize it or not, they will look at food a little differently, maybe while food shopping or maybe by paying more attention to how they feel. One story plants a seed, and that seed will grow with more time and by hearing more stories. That seed will grow every time that person eats whole, real, not-modified food and feels better. Then that person will one day share their story, and around and around we go. Let me sum it up in one sentence: a plant-based diet with zero processed foods healed my psoriasis after having it for almost twenty years. As a result, I'm with my teacher, Joshua Rosenthal, who said GMOs do not have a place in our food, body, or planet, and I couldn't agree more!

Now that I have gotten that off my chest and shared more valuable information with you, back to my meals…

If it is mid-morning or I am running late for lunch, I make sure I have a handful of mixed nuts (brazil, almond, hazel, pecans), an apple with almond butter, and carrots or celery dipped in hummus. Sometimes, I make kale chips, dried fruit, homemade granola bars and cookies made from oats, almond flour, fruit, and nuts. I also love picking up some healthy raw snacks from the health food store to have on hand. If you were hungry at my old job and asked anyone for food, they would all point you in my direction! I had a drawer filled with goodies as well as a shelf I shared with a co-worker. No one was going hungry if I could help it, and if they needed a snack, they were going to eat a healthy snack! I totally get this personality trait from my dad; it made him so happy to feed people and watch them enjoy themselves. Food really can be love, as long as it's real food.

I used to always bring a prepared lunch to work and eat it at my desk. Unfortunately, working in television, this is the norm because there was never time to go out and relax while eating. Please understand that I don't ever recommend eating while working because we all should eat and digest our food in a relaxed state and environment, but trust me, I've been there and lived that fast-paced life for years. My regular lunch on the starter cleanse was a salad with tons of veggies, nuts, and seeds, and olive oil, lemon, and sea salt for dressing. Sometimes, I'd have a veggie burger on top, depending on the ingredients, or I'd throw on beans or a piece of salmon. Salmon was the only protein (versus animal protein) I'd make an exception for because I knew my skin liked it. I also made sautéed veggies with brown rice and avocado. Sometimes, I'd add black beans. To this day, this is my staple lunch, which I've been making about three times a week for what feels like forever. The great news is I think anything with avocado on top is delicious. Add a little olive oil and sea salt, and that's what I call my yum! When I worked in the city, I kept a large jar of olive oil and sea salt at my desk. Sometimes, I'd shake it up and buy mixed greens from a nearby place that had tons of healthy raw options. I'd also make interesting vegan dishes, like faux mac and cheese and tons of other dishes I'd found in numerous books and online. It's amazing what's out there! Once you get the hang of this new lifestyle and the ingredients you can use, searching for a special recipe or meal can be fun.[21]

Snacks at any point during the day in cleanse mode were usually fruit and nuts and pretty much anything I've already listed. Your goal is never to leave yourself so hungry that you make a bad choice because you are in a rush and just need to eat something.

In those early stages of eating cleaner and greener, dinner was usually vegetables, salmon, quinoa or, again, a recipe I found such as a butternut squash soup or something. There are tons of choices. (Don't forget to check out my website for a list of great books that are not only inspiring to read but have wonderful recipes in them, too.) All I have to say is thank heavens for vegan recipes! Just so you know, my Ps diet isn't really a vegan lifestyle because 20 percent of the time you can eat fish (no shellfish), poultry, or lamb, as per Dr. Pagano. But vegan recipes tend to use the ingredients you can have, so it makes life easier. One thing I learned early on was to swap regular dairy milk for almond milk or coconut milk. I know how hard this could be for people, especially being set in your ways for most of your life, but I find it's not that hard when your goal of healing is the priority. Almond milk and coconut milk make wonderful smoothies and even "ice cream." The hardest part for me, initially, was making the time to prepare and cook, but I enjoy preparing food now, and it helps that I have never felt healthier!

On weekends, I would let myself have eggs for breakfast, and it didn't seem to hinder my progress, so that was great. Everyone is different, though. I appreciated that food break and didn't splurge on eggs more than twice a week. If you are concerned that you might have an allergy to eggs, then, of course, stay away from them.

---

21   Some of these recipes on my site: http://www.healingmyskin.com.

Another important step is keeping hydrated throughout the day. Think about it this way: if the amount of water in our bodies is between 50-75 percent, as adults, how much water do you need to consume each day to stay hydrated? Many experts recommend at least eight eight-ounce glasses. The Global Healing Center, a group that develops and sells the highest quality organic health products, explains how we need to drink enough water to flush the kidneys or liver to allow the colon to move our bowels.[22] If we don't do this, we allow our bodies to retain the unhealthy toxins, and if they stay put for too long, they will get reabsorbed into our bloodstream and circulate those harmful chemicals to every organ in our bodies. By the way, when I say water, I don't mean flavored water or water with added powders like those "diet light" ones, which are just extra chemicals, I mean filtered healthy water.

A teacher of mine once said, "Whatever you do, don't drink tap water." He didn't elaborate, but from my research, I'm pretty sure he was referring to all the chemicals it's treated with to kill bacteria. Depending where you are, some sources have been found to contain arsenic and other pollutants such as fluoride, chlorine, bacteria, and pesticides. I don't know about you, but when I read this, it made me never want to drink tap water again! One would think bottled water is safer, but according to the Environmental Protection Agency, bottled water may be expected to contain at least small amounts of some contaminants. Also, chemicals are used to make the plastic into its shape and add flexibility, and these chemicals can leach into the water you drink.

So, what do we do? We need to find a way to alkalize our drinking water and remove the impurities. I started off by

---

22   http://www.globalhealingcenter.com.

buying the pH drops they sell at health food stores or online, but they are expensive and, to be honest, I found it a bit frustrating to carry them around with me at all times to put in my water when I went out to eat or was walking around. It was fine when I was at work sitting at my desk all day with a glass of water, but other times I'd forget, or I'd use it all up pretty quickly. There are alkalizing powders, but they felt inconvenient too. I used a Britta filter for years, but never realized it wasn't alkalizing my water, only removing some of the who-knows-what. Plus, the filter replacements were expensive. The ultimate solution was an Apex alkaline water filter ($100 on Amazon), which attaches to my kitchen sink. It has a filtration system that alkalizes your tap water while removing impurities. It attaches pretty easily, and there are five stages of filtration that remove heavy metals, chlorine, microorganisms, and odor while adding minerals such as calcium, magnesium, and potassium. Alkaline water helps prevent aging and diseases, so anything we can do helps. There are a plethora of filter systems online, just be sure to read the reviews and buy the best one. I know $100 seems like a lot, but the filter doesn't need to be replaced for twelve months and, to me, that's totally worth it. Buy yourself some safe non-leaching plastic containers and you can bring your healthy water wherever you go. I recently purchased a glass bottle from a company called CamelBak, and it's great. It's not as heavy as I thought it would be and it's protected in a silicone sleeve in case you drop it.

Also, please keep in mind that coffee is not a water replacement. If you are a coffee drinker and waking up without it means not ever wanting to wake up at all, there are some wonderful replacements out there that can take its place. Are they coffee? No. Do they taste exactly like coffee? No. But I must say, when I drink them, I get my "coffee fix," and everyone I have recommended them to feels the same way, or at least they say they enjoy them. So if coffee is the hardest thing for you to give up (it was for me!), I strongly suggest you try these alternatives. Even though Dr. Pagano doesn't say you have to, from my experience giving up coffee truly did help heal my skin. Maybe that was because I was drinking multiple cups a day, so between the caffeine and acidity, it majorly irritated my gut and my skin.

I have to say I loved nothing more than walking down the streets of Manhattan on my way to work with a creamy latte in hand. I used to leave extra early to walk a few subway stations further every morning to add in a little walking, and the first thing I did was stop at a coffee shop. It was habitual to walk everywhere with coffee in hand. I loved it. It comforted me in a way I can't describe. It made me feel complete. I thoroughly enjoyed sipping it on a nice, cold winter's day while walking along. It was my friend, or so I thought. As soon as I quit, I noticed the headaches I'd gotten for years vanished and my skin clearing accelerated. I'm not promising this will happen for you, but I do know that caffeine is a gut irritant, and I can imagine you will feel something good once you are past the withdrawal stage. My advice is to mix it up. Have your cup of coffee and, instead of a second cup, try one of the alternatives. You might just like it.

For coffee replacements here are some wonderful options that have zero acidity and are caffeine free:

- Teeccino Herbal Coffee, made with organic carob, chicory, dandelion, dates, figs, and, depending on which flavor you get, some have almonds, hazelnuts, or vanilla.

- Dandy Blend, made from extracts of roasted barley, rye, chicory root, dandelion root and sugar beetroot. The great thing about Dandy Blend is it also comes in these little packets of instant powder, that you can drink hot or cold. I add four drops of liquid stevia (English toffee flavored) and a dash of cinnamon. It tastes very similar to coffee, believe it or not, and I know of people who drink it black and love it. Some people even report a slight surge in energy like with caffeine but without the dive later.

You can find both of these online or in your local health food store. I buy mine from Amazon. I like to add a dash of almond or coconut milk and cinnamon; it tastes fantastic this way.

Another thing that helped me in the very beginning before I discovered these two options was decaffeinated chai. I would add hot water, almond milk, and a dash of cinnamon and, wow, does it ever quench my sweet-tooth and coffee cravings. The great news is, with decaf chai and even some of the iced herbal teas, you can go to Starbucks with your friends! When you order a decaf chai, you have to say teabag or they will give you a latte which has lots of sugar. It's called Chai Tea Misto and is great with steamed coconut milk. I add a dash of cinnamon, and it does brighten my day. The most important piece to remember is you must be prepared for those cravings ahead of time and have some go to replacements that are enjoyable enough to satiate your desire for the real thing.

Along with the above replacements, there are also special teas that Dr. Pagano strongly suggests you drink every day to clean out your intestines and thicken your intestinal walls.

These are American yellow saffron tea and slippery elm bark tea. You can get these from the Heritage Store (heritagestore. com) or most health food stores. They aren't the cheapest, but one bag of each will last you a very long time; so trust me, you are getting your money's worth. You are only using a quarter teaspoon at a time and drinking it once a day. Just be sure to drink them ten to twelve hours apart. The saffron tea acts as an antiseptic, cleaning out your intestines, while the slippery elm coats and thickens your intestinal walls to prevent stuff from passing through. I like to drink the saffron in the morning and the elm at night.

The saffron tastes very similar to chamomile tea, in my opinion, not strong or bad at all. The slippery elm tea is a different story. You mix it with cold water, not hot; and be sure to follow the instructions on the bag because it says to wait ten minutes before drinking it, then to drink it quickly before it thickens. It's not the most pleasant taste. I don't like it or hate it, but I do drink it quickly to get it over with, whereas I have friends who can't stomach it. Luckily, it comes in other forms now, including liquid drops and even cough drops that you can suck on that don't taste too bad. The cough drops taste a bit bland and chalky — nothing you would suck on for enjoyment, but not as bad as the powdered tea. The liquid drops aren't as bad either; again, it's not something you want to drink, but you try it because you try anything that will help heal your skin. I've bought both of these forms from health food stores, Whole Foods, or Amazon. As I said above, any form of slippery elm will thicken your intestinal walls, and that's what you want, so toxins don't continue to seep through. I drank these teas every day, and I believe they played a huge part in my healing.

On top of changing my diet drastically and drinking these teas, I was already juicing vegetables and fruits, and taking a slew of vitamins such as vitamin D, B, omega-3, blue-green algae, and kelp. My vitamin regimen is different today. Now, I take a probiotic, multi-vitamin, and omega-3 fish oil (made from whole, not synthetic, foods). I take these per the instructions of my nutritional practitioner who I see every few months. I recommend you find a health practitioner or an understanding doctor to figure out what supplements your body needs. The two companies I get my supplements from are Premier Research Labs and Standard Process. I get my fish oil vitamins from Nordic Naturals.

⋑

Now, as promised, for some disaster stories to put a smile on your face and prove, once again, I'm human. Let's start with juicing recipe disasters. When you start to dabble in the kitchen, there's no doubt you will mess up and find yourself sadly standing over the trash bin saying goodbye to whatever it was you just tried to make and failed. In the trash go your hard-earned money, time, and nutritious food. It's a very disappointing feeling, and I know it all too well. This will happen to you. Take it as one of those learning lessons in life we wish we could do without. My problem is that I try to get creative and veer away from the original recipe. Don't do it! Unless you are like my friend Suzi, who calls herself the iron chef; she can't follow a recipe to save her life, yet everything she touches in the kitchen turns to (delicious) gold! We can't all be like Suzi, so until you get more comfortable in the kitchen, follow the recipe! Trust that they are published for a reason and that the creator already went through many failed attempts to get it perfect for you.

Since I tend to become incredibly courageous when juicing, I know some of you reading this book will not relate to my juicing woes. My hope is, one day, you will. Juicing has helped heal my life in so many ways, and I know it will heal yours too. I've been juicing for a long time, and I'm at a point now where I just throw in everything from the bottom refrigerator drawer, plus the proverbial kitchen sink. Sometimes, my husband looks at me funny and asks, "What's in this? Why does it look like mud?" My reply is always, "Just drink it; you need your greens!"

The two mistakes I'll never experiment with again are garlic and oranges. Yes, you read that right, I said garlic. Juicing garlic sounds gross, I know. I juice garlic along with other fruits and veggies when I get sick. Garlic is known to fight sickness, especially the common cold. It has a ridiculous amount of nutrients in it, and I've even read that it has almost every nutrient your body needs. One lesson I learned really quickly is not to juice an entire clove in one glass of juice. I don't know how I got that down without vomiting, and I stank for days. In this case, less is more. Lesson learned!

The lesson I learned when juicing oranges is to remove the outer peel. It ruined my juice with the most bitter, awful taste, and it saddened me to see all the rest of the organic fruits and veggies in that juice get poured down the drain. It's too bad because orange peels contain healthy essential oils our bodies appreciate. There are plenty of other uses for those orange peels, but I would suggest keeping them out of your juice!

As for cooking disasters, I'll never forget the first meal I cooked for Mike in our new apartment after living together for all of five days; and I assure you he will never let me forget it either! It's our inside joke about oregano, forever and ever, until death do us part.

I decided to make our first meal in the apartment a healthier version of chicken parmesan by using almond flour mixed with herbs and spices instead of bread crumbs (which have sugar, gluten, preservatives, etc.). I was making two versions, one batch for me (plain), and one batch for Mike (with tomato sauce and cheese). I started by following the recipe, and then I'm not quite sure what happened after that; I just know I wanted to improvise and make a very tasty almond bread crumb mix! There seemed to be too much almond flour and not enough herbs and spices, so I used a tablespoon of oregano in the flour mix as well as a tablespoon in the tomato sauce. You guessed it, way too much oregano!

We were very excited about trying it, and while chewing our first bite, our first impressions were that it wasn't so bad compared to using bread crumbs. We both thought there was a bit too much oregano, but it didn't stop us from having a piece each. The next day we were unpacking and getting ready to go to Ikea. We decided to have the leftovers for lunch before leaving. Now, I don't know what happened overnight; maybe the oregano had babies, and those babies had babies. I don't know! But, eating it the next day was utterly impossible. We both took a few bites while looking at each other in horror.

Mike told me later he finished half a piece because he didn't want me to feel bad because I had tried to make this nice meal in our new home. By the time we were in the car traveling to Ikea, Mike had turned to me and said he didn't feel well, that he thought he might need to throw up. He started burping to relieve himself and said with this disgusted look on his face, "I'm burping up oregano."

I replied, "There are two tablespoons of it in your belly!"

We started cracking up so hard we were crying! It's too bad because I read that only half a teaspoon has the antioxidant power of three cups of raw spinach. Unfortunately, we just can't find it in ourselves to eat it anymore and if we do it has to be very little. The point of my story? Follow the recipe! I have learned my lesson that less is more — which has become Mike's favorite saying and what he says to me every time I'm cooking; it's very annoying but cute!

Hopefully, your tummy won't be too upset with you during this time of trying new things and messing up good recipes. In case it comes in handy for you, my go-to for helping soothe my stomach after an episode like the one above is mint. I like to simmer a few sprigs in boiling water and then sip it. It helps with everything digestion: gas, bloating, heartburn, diarrhea, constipation; basically, any gastrointestinal issues. Two other great choices to help soothe your tummy are peppermint and ginger tea. I buy both by the box, and I also like to use fresh ginger. I'll cut a small piece off, remove the skin, and throw it in some hot water. It's always very calming and makes me feel better!

Before I get to the after-dinner treats allowed on the starter cleanse, I wanted to share one more major event that was life-changing and helped me see what happens when we get ready for a big trip or a vacation and want to go live-it-up. I'm adding it here because it also has a little lesson about those "sweet things" that are hard to give up. Although I discuss this from an emotional aspect in a later chapter, I wanted to share what happens when you travel, have Ps, and want to treat yourself to everything in sight.

A few summers ago, I went to Ireland for my sister's wedding. It is a beautiful country, and it was quite a unique and incredible wedding. I had been Ps free at the time because it was after my very first healing journey. Usually, when I travel, I like to have the attitude of "when in Rome" as far as food and beverages go. I look at it this way: this is most likely the only time I will visit this part of the world, and I want to get the full experience and fully take in the culture. So in Ireland, my attitude was "Bring on the meat, potatoes, and Guinness!" Oh, and what delicious Guinness it was. I'm not even a fan of it here in the States, but over there it was just so delicious.

While I was consuming those three things all week, I couldn't help but think about how much of it was going to push my Ps to rear its ugly head again, but I guess a part of me was curious to learn what it would really take? Would it take a burger? A steak? A steak, potatoes, and three glasses of wine? How much acidic stuff could I get away with consuming before I saw the negative effects? I had not touched anything too acidic for almost a year, and my skin had cleared 95 percent, so I found myself thinking these crazy thoughts while traveling like how much time did I have before an outbreak? As if my life was going to end or, worse, I would be covered in patchy red scales!

For almost a year on my strict health journey, I thought every second about what I was going to put in my mouth and it was exhausting. All that thinking and paying attention to and planning; so I was tired, and I felt I deserved a break. I wanted to eat cheese. I wanted that cupcake at the work birthday parties. I wanted to enjoy a glass of wine with dinner. I wanted to enjoy my nightshades without the side of fear or guilt. I liked not having to think about what to get for lunch and just grab a sandwich from the deli on busy days. There were so many little things I missed having the freedom to do.

In Ireland, if I wanted a dessert after dinner, I was going to have a dessert after dinner. And what dessert is not full of sugar? Ironically, sugar is not this terrible thing people make it out to be because our bodies actually need sugar; it's the *type* we use that is the problem. Our cells use sugar as its main source of energy and to motivate the pancreas to do its job, which is to produce insulin. What I'm talking about is glucose, a simple sugar that our bodies process. Now, refined white table sugar is sugar that has been processed and stripped of all of its nutrients, and that is what not only has a bad rap but is downright dangerous to our health since our bodies can't easily process it. If you eat refined sugar daily, it overloads the liver, whose job it is to store excess sugar. The liver now has no choice but to expand, and when it reaches its maximum capacity, the excess sugar is turned into fatty acids and deposited into other parts of our bodies. Think about where you gain weight—what are your problem areas? For me, it's my middle bits: hips, stomach, and thighs. I'm sure every woman reading this can relate. Some of this fat even remains in the liver, causing fatty liver disease, which can cause all sorts of other medical problems down the road.

Sugar is also very addictive and has been proven to be more addictive than cocaine. Crazy, right? In studies where mice had a choice of sugar versus cocaine, they picked sugar. When we eat cookies and cake, it causes a release of dopamine, which is a chemical in our brain that helps us feel happy. When we eat fruit made from natural sugar that is loaded with nutrients, the dopamine release isn't as large, so it just doesn't satisfy us in the same way. This is why we seek out the foods with refined sugars so often: because we want those positive feelings again. Also, something else to keep in mind: we often allow that positive, happy feeling to override the "I'm full" feeling. Now we have an even bigger problem: overeating, indulging in nutrition-less foods and gaining weight. This is why our country has an obesity epidemic on its hands. In some ways, we really shouldn't blame ourselves for craving sweets all the time. Imagine, it's almost like we are being drugged. Look at all the sugar we consume in our food, our sodas, even in our bread, and of course, in our treats.

I never realized how evil sugar could be until I removed all the processed refined sugar from my diet. I couldn't believe what I was seeing. My Ps slowly faded a little bit every day, right before my eyes. I also noticed my constant headaches vanished, and I felt more clarity and energy. The foods I removed were bread, bagels, croissants, cookies, cake, chips, crackers, white pasta, etc. Trust me, it wasn't easy. Over time — and I mean a lot of time — I discovered some wonderful substitutes so I could still enjoy a bowl of pasta or a cookie or toast. It takes time and patience, and I am trying to help you skip a step to get healed more quickly than I did. Weaning off sugar is best done in baby steps. My main source of sugar now is fruit, and I've gotten so used to it that when I do have a piece of cake or cookies they taste incredibly sweet to me — too sweet, really.

The side effects from refined sugars include obesity, heart disease, cancer, poor cognitive functioning, tooth decay, diabetes, fatty liver disease, digestive issues, auto-immune diseases, and the list goes on. On this journey, I've discovered I have a bit of an addiction to sugar, a sweet tooth, above the refined type even to the healthier alternatives that are loaded with nutrients. I never thought I could have an addiction since I use the natural replacements, the ones that come from

Mother Earth, like trees and plants. But my day doesn't seem complete without a little sweetness, so I have to monitor it. For example, I don't go overboard and sit with a big bowl of dried fruit while watching a movie or anything like that. I don't eat dates, then guzzle some maple syrup, and finish it off with raw honey, either. I just slowly realized that I need that little "sweet cap" and decided that, if that was my addiction, and that I've been like that my entire life (probably because my mom always had cake and cookies in the house growing up), I would honor it but keep it in check.

I'm pretty certain that most people have a sugar addiction and just don't know it. Sugar is not just cake and cookies; it's everything processed, like chips and bread. Think about that burger and fries you eat when you go out or that sandwich you take to work—sugar is everywhere, in everything, so it is important to start to pay attention now.

As a test one time, my sister and I agreed to do an experiment and cut sugar out completely for three days to see how hard it would be. My poor sister went through major withdrawal, which left her with a two-week-long headache. My experience was not as bad, but I was also more used to eating healthier with veggies, healthy protein, legumes, nuts, and seeds than she was. My sister gave up sandwiches, granola bars, and chips, and that wasn't easy. It was a fascinating learning lesson for both of us.

Because fruit is not the only source of sugar, the natural sweeteners I use instead, that at least give my body some antioxidants, are terrific replacements but need to be used in moderation and are as follows:

- **Dates:** These are by far my favorite! I love eating them plain when I need something sweet. I also put them in my smoothies and cookies, and when I'm making homemade almond milk. One date perfectly sweetens it slightly. You can even make a date paste to smear on toast or use in baking desserts. They are packed with copper, potassium, iron, magnesium, and vitamin B6. They are easily digested, can lower cholesterol, and re- duce the risk of stroke.

- **Raw honey**: This is another one of my favorites. Honey is jam-packed with essential nutrients, like iron, vita- min B6, and potassium, that help the growth of healthy bacteria in our guts. I use this in my baking as well as when I'm going on a long run. I'll carry a bit with me for a little energy when I desperately need it. (Not that I run long distances often.) Also, know that honey in its raw form has way more benefits than after it is pas- teurized. So buy raw whenever possible.

- **Stevia**: Stevia is from a plant from South America that is related to the sunflower. It's much sweeter than sugar—a lot sweeter—and some people find it has a chemical-like aftertaste, but I don't mind it. My favor- ite brands are Sweetleaf and Stevia in the Raw, but there are a few other really good ones, such as Pure or NuNaturals. When you shop for stevia be sure to read the label to make sure it doesn't contain any fill- ers and additives like dextrose or maltodextrin. It even promotes healthy blood sugar levels and weight loss. I love putting one or two drops in certain teas if I'm craving a little sweetness. I also use it when I make my hubby yogurt. For a healthier, quick yogurt, I'll buy plain grass-fed yogurt and mix it with half a packet of stevia and add cut-up banana or berries. This way you have a healthy probiotic with four times less sugar.

- **Coconut sugar:** I'm all about everything coconut! I love fresh coconut meat, coconut water, and coconut milk. I recently learned about coconut sugar from my cousin. She swears by it; it's all she uses. The more research I did on it, the more I liked what I was reading. It's loaded with nutrients like iron, zinc, and calcium, just to name a few. You can find a cupcake recipe that uses it on the freebies page of my website. It's delicious, and I now use it in a lot of my baking. It's very light and doesn't make the desserts taste too sweet.

- **Maple syrup:** I use this in my cookies sometimes and love it. Who knew that this real (not the corn starch and food coloring) syrup we love on our pancakes is rich in antioxidants and helps neutralize free radicals in our bodies? It is a wonderful source of manganese and contains calcium, potassium, and zinc. I've read that Grade B contains more beneficial antioxidants, so if you have a choice between A and B, choose B!

- **Brown rice syrup:** I use this syrup when I make these amazing brown rice crispy treats recipe found in Alicia Silverstone's book, *The Kind Diet*. You can also use it in baking cookies or making granola bars. The fermenting process brown rice goes through to become a sweet syrup helps break down the sugars, so they are easily digestible. This process is key. The rice is fermented with enzymes that break down its starch.

Now that I'm craving something sweet from writing about all this, I hope that my digression helps you learn there are so many other great ways to make a sweet tooth happy and to enjoy a treat after dinner. But, before completely moving on and to finish my Ireland story, the trip was fabulous even though every food I consumed eventually stepped up to greet me later. Yes, you guessed it, my Ps came back with a vengeance. So, just like you, I was forced to go back to the beginning with my starter cleanse, and now I know that when I travel my indulgences can no longer be anything and everything.

Getting back to my initial cleanse schedule: After dinner, if at home, I would make some herbal tea or even indulge in a little fruit or a raw dessert from a nearby vegan restaurant. Not a normal white sugary dessert, but something made from fruits, nuts, and nut flours. I now make vegan almond flour and rolled oat cookies with carob chips, and they are hands down better than any chocolate chip cookie I've ever tasted. When out for dinner, I'd always have some herbal tea while my friends would sip their wine or coffee.

Planning ahead is definitely one of the necessities of the program. For example, there were some nights I would have to plan around my exercise schedule, like Tuesdays when I'd go to an early evening yoga class after work. I would make sure to bring some extra food to eat at the end of the day while I was still at work. Otherwise, I'd be too starving by class time to do yoga and would risk indulging in the wrong foods.

I also used to see a personal trainer back then, so I'd always make sure I had something to eat or even a smoothie a few hours beforehand. My lifestyle today compared to five years ago is very different. Back then, I was working full time in TV, living in New York City, and single. I only had me and Max to worry about. Today, I'm married, living in the suburbs, and working from home and commuting to the city part time. My life has changed between finding love, finding my purpose to help people, and discovering the importance of self-love. My classes at the Institute for Integrative Nutrition also kept me busy learning as they taught us over a hundred different dietary theories, so we students naturally experimented to find what worked best for us so we could teach our clients to do the same. And so you know, I realized quickly that a 100 percent plant-based diet is not for me, but 90/10 is. It's what I can stick with and even enjoy.

After the rigid starter cleanse, which you should remain on as long as it takes to clear your skin, you can start slowly to add back certain foods to see what works for you. I now follow the 90/10 diet created by my teacher Joshua Rosenthal. Ninety percent of the time, I do the best I can and 10 percent of the time, I eat whatever I want. I find that this is the first lifestyle choice regarding diet I've made that works for me. Now, once a week or on a weekend, when I am at a bar or restaurant and indulge in some pub food, I don't beat myself up for enjoying that one meal. That being said, it never ends up being as good as I was expecting and I prefer a yummy healthy meal any day.

As you can see, any new process is hard, and it does take work, but soon you will see a little difference on your skin, and that will keep you incredibly motivated. I missed so many things initially, mostly the coffee, but going for meals with friends wasn't as hard as I thought it might be. I would try to plan some dinners at vegan or vegetarian restaurants, but I did find most places have some vegetables or salad. Hopefully, they had a piece of chicken or fish too. Sometimes, I was in a situation where I was invited to an event and I didn't have many choices, or it was impossible to skip on anything cooked in butter or oils. When faced with this occasional situation that I truly had no control over, I just ate as well as I could, let it go, and enjoyed myself.

Don't get me wrong; today this is still something I have to work on consistently. Life is busy, and there will always be travel, parties, events, and such. I'm a bit less strict these days when I'm in a situation where I'm surrounded by foods I don't normally eat, only because I know very well what my body needs and can nourish myself with whole foods the rest of the time. If I'm traveling for the weekend to a place where I can't shop and cook, I'll do the best I can. I'm also learning to release the guilt little by little. When I travel abroad, my "when in Rome" philosophy is a little less indulgent, but if it means I eat a pork shank in Germany, so be it. I love traveling; it's very important to me, so I choose to live and let go during those times. And I no longer feel the need to sample *all* of the local delicacies, because I choose my health first.

As I've mentioned, I've learned over the years what works for my body, and that is the 90/10 diet. That works for me. If I were still covered in Ps, it would be a different story. I would be 100 percent doing the best I can. At the beginning of my journey, I was covered with spots on my legs and elbows. Today I am not. I'll get a few spots here or there when I am stressed, not taking care of myself, and eating poorly. I know what needs to be done to make those spots fade away. I need to eat clean, meditate, work less, laugh more, and love myself. The phrase "I am in control" is a constant reminder and something I want you to start saying to yourself every day. To help you see how you can move from a cleanse to a lifetime of eating in control — because eating cleaner does mean eating greener — here is a summary of what foods I eat today:

- **All fruit and veggies, aside from the nightshades**: These give our bodies the nutrients they need to thrive.

- **Whole grains**: Brown rice, buckwheat, oats, and such. They provide fiber (among other things) and give you energy to stay alive.
- **Beans and legumes:** Black beans, pinto beans, kidney beans, chickpeas, lentils, etc. These are a wonderful protein source, provide tons of fiber, are filling, and keep you going all day; they are great for your digestion, regulate your blood sugar, lower cholesterol, and help prevent heart disease.
- **Nuts**: Raw almonds, pecans, brazil, hazelnuts, cashews, including nut butters and nut flours to bake with. Nuts are a great protein source, lower cholesterol, fight inflammation, contain fiber, and protect us from cancer.
- **Seeds:** Quinoa, chia, hemp, flax, etc. Seeds offer all sorts of vitamins we need such as vitamin E, essential amino acids, and magnesium; they also have fiber, antioxidants, and omegas. In case you didn't know, chia seeds are little miracles of their own and have a powerful nutritional punch. (I put them in my smoothie every day.) A one ounce (28 grams or 2 tablespoons) serving of chia seeds contains:
  - Fiber: 11 grams;
  - Protein: 4 grams;
  - Fat: 9 grams (5 of which are omega-3s);
  - Calcium: 18 percent of the RDA (recommended daily allowance);
  - Manganese: 30 percent of the RDA;
  - Magnesium: 30 percent of the RDA;
  - Phosphorus: 27 percent of the RDA;
  - They also contain a decent amount of zinc, vitamin B3 (niacin), potassium, vitamin B1 (thiamine) and vitamin B2.[23]

---

23   https://authoritynutrition.com/11-proven-health-benefits-of-chia-seeds/.

- **Animal protein (sparingly)**: I limit this to organic, cage-free, non-GMO chicken and wild salmon.
- **Oils from plants or nuts/seeds**: This includes extra virgin olive, coconut, avocado, walnut, sesame, or almond oil.
- **Sugars**: Raw honey, organic maple syrup, stevia, agave, coconut sugar, palm sugar. (Again, use sparingly, because it's still sugar!)
- **Dairy substitutes**: Almond milk, coconut milk, brazil nut milk, cashew milk, or even flax milk if you are concerned about allergies.

There is a lot of variety in the above list, and you will be surprised how much can be done with them.

Then there are the foods I avoid: Red meat, white refined sugar, dairy, processed food, and nightshade veggies.

Now that I am working from home and my schedule has changed, I also wanted to share what my day looks like on a 24-hour schedule:

6:30 a.m.: I wake up and first thing I do after saying goodbye to my hubby as he leaves for work is to meditate. I lie back in bed for ten minutes while I listen to a soft YouTube meditation music video. (If I'm planning a long walk, I skip this meditation, knowing my walk will be my meditation.) Then I prepare my hot water with lemon and sip it while I get dressed. While I get dressed, I say "I love you" in the mirror a few times. When I apply coconut oil on my skin, I thank it and express loving thoughts for all it does for me.

7:30 a.m.: Then I make juice or a smoothie for my first breakfast. My latest smoothie I'm obsessed with is spinach, almond milk, chia seeds, banana, strawberries, and blueberries.

8:30 a.m.: I exercise, which for me is either a long walk, a run, or a cardio class at the gym. I usually walk every day, whether it's a mile to get to the train station when I need to go into the city, or just to cool down after running or being at the gym. My walks have truly become special meditation moments for me. I take in the birds, the trees, the flowers, the beautiful homes, the breeze, and the sun. I feel more present and out of my thoughts the most when I'm walking.

9:30 a.m.: I shower, and when I'm in the shower I take this opportunity to meditate for a few minutes right before I get out. I make the water a little hotter and stand there just feeling it on my back. I say the following affirmations: "I love and approve of myself," "I deserve the very best in life," and "I am alive to all the joys of living." I got these affirmations from Louise Hay's book *Heal Your Body*. According to Louise, both the good in our lives as well as the *dis-eases* are the results of thought patterns that form our experiences. She believes psoriasis is a manifestation of the fear of being hurt, deadening the sense of the self, and refusing to accept responsibility for our feelings. These are affirmations she suggests we say every day. I love her work, and I, too, believe a lot of our illnesses manifest from negative thinking. I believe these affirmations have brought beautiful yet subtle changes into my life and skin.

10:00 a.m.: Breakfast #2. Usually, I'm hungry when I return from working out, so these are my go-tos for breakfast: Ezekiel toast with almond butter and berries; coconut milk yogurt with berries, nuts, and seeds; a small bowl of fruit with various nuts; or chia pudding with berries. (The chia pudding recipe is on my website; it won't disappoint!)

10:30 a.m.: I start my day. Lately, it's been a lot of writing! I'm also working on my business, Healing My Skin, which I recently launched. The months previous had been over-booked with finishing my certification, a lot of health coaching, studying, homework, and test-taking.

11:30 a.m.: Snack time (if I'm hungry). This usually consists of a piece of fruit with nuts if I didn't have them for breakfast. I love nothing more than a small bowl of blackberries, blueberries, raspberries, and a mix of almonds, pecans, Brazil, and macadamia nuts. It's become my favorite little snack. I also make healthy cookies or banana bread, so if something is made, I may have a piece of that.

1:30 p.m.: Lunch is usually veggies and tofu. I'm in love with my new Vegetti maker, which turns veggies like zucchini into noodles. I'll sprinkle that with olive oil, garlic, and sea salt, and it's fantastic. I'll sauté tofu and broccoli or kale. I love organic firm tofu from Trader Joe's. Sometimes I'll make a salad with mixed greens, cucumber, endives, carrots, chickpeas, avocado, and hemp seeds; it depends on what I have in the house.

Sometimes I'll eat organic chicken, turkey or wild caught salmon when my body craves it. I am not a vegan or a vegetarian by any means. My lifestyle is very different now. I listen to my body and give it what it wants.

6:00 p.m.: Dinner is always veggies! Veggies with soup, veggie burger, turkey burger, salmon, salad, sweet potato fries, tofu, brown rice or quinoa pasta, or whole grains like brown rice or quinoa. If I'm out to eat, I'll order chicken or fish with veggies or a big healthy salad with all sorts of yummy toppings like nuts, dried fruit, seeds, beans, etc.

Evening: I'll end my day with some relaxation time in the evening, talking with my hubby while sipping a nice hot mug of Dandy Blend, decaf chai tea, or Teeccino Herbal Coffee with a little almond milk and cinnamon. I don't find myself eating dessert these days, but if I feel the desire to, I'll have some fruit. Frozen grapes or blueberries are surprisingly delicious, by the way! Also, a wonderful dessert is banana ice cream made from two frozen bananas, 1/3 cup of almond milk, and two tablespoons of walnuts. You just blend it up, and it really tastes like ice cream! You can add frozen strawberries too! (Thanks to Dr. Joel Fuhrman for that idea! He has a bunch of other raw healthy desserts in his book, *Eat to Live*.)

Not every day looks like the one above. Sometimes I work in the city and am gone from 8:00 a.m. until 8:00 p.m., so I need to prepare my meals and bring them with me. As a free-lancer, I move around from job to job, so I'll actually bring a backpack of food with me. I'm aware most people are not willing to go to these lengths, but when you are on a mission to heal, you will do what you have to. It is very important to me to know what I'm putting into my body. Here and there I'd buy lunch from healthy cafés and am very lucky to work in a city that has a plethora of them!

Ever since I learned about primary food at the Institute for Integrative Nutrition—which means relationships, career, money, exercise, stress, spiritual practice—my whole world has changed. I want to find balance in my life with every-thing. I want my relationship with my hubby to be healthy and strong. I want to surround myself with only positive people. I want eight hours of sleep. I want to feed my body food that nourishes me. I want to work on my emotional and spiritual life by meditating, writing, walking, and being more present. I want to have a healthy and loving relationship with money. And I want to keep stress out of my life as much as possible.

My whole life I've always been on the go: stressed out, rushing, commuting, working hard, and feeling time wasn't on my side. The environment in TV and film production is anything but calm. Now, all I want to do is take my time, keep stress to a minimum, work on my schedule doing what I'm passionate about, and take care of my health. I've been happi-est since this new chapter of my life, where my health comes first, and I don't do anything before starting my day off in a way that serves to replenish my body and soul.

I hope these little stories and the rundown of food help you commit to drinking lemon in hot water in the morning, doing some juicing, picking some new go-to foods, doing your best to go organic (at least from the Dirty Dozen list), and staying away from GMO food. So go ahead and go into your kitchen and get rid of the "killer" foods and introduce the healthy ones. Stop yourself from eating when in a rush or starved or simply have "that craving," because you would have to leave the house to get it, and let the craving pass you by. There is a good chance it will.

All of these basic foods will help move your body from acidic to alkaline. Also, they are all anti-inflammatory. What I mean by that is they help reduce inflammation, which then helps you heal. Inflammation is now known to be a silent killer. We all know what good inflammation is, right? We get a cut or a scrape, and next thing you know, it's red and swollen because white blood cells are rushing to the scene to kill the bad bacteria and protect you from infection. This is acute inflammation; it lasts for hours or days and is part of the body's immune defense. You have to love the way our bodies know what to do; it's simply incredible!

Chronic inflammation is what I'm referring to, which lasts in our bodies for years. It's what happens when we are constantly putting our immune system under attack by bombarding it with inflammatory foods, lack of sleep, or stress. Chronic inflammation is known to play a huge part in diseases including cancer, heart disease, auto-immune, and asthma. It wasn't until I stopped putting acidic foods that create inflammation in my body that I started to heal.

Some of the top inflammatory foods are sugar, fried foods, refined flour, dairy, synthetic sweeteners, processed foods with artificial additives and coloring, and saturated fats. In 2012, in only a few months after removing these foods, I watched my Ps slowly disappear before my eyes. My elbows looked like normal elbows. No more did I feel insecure wearing t-shirts! No more was I insecure when a person's hand went to grab the back of my arm when talking to me in a loud bar. (This tended to happen a lot.) I wasn't used to this clear skin at all, by the way. I found myself at work checking my elbows in the bathroom mirror to make sure it hadn't appeared all of a sudden. It felt too good to be true.

I want to help sufferers of this devastating skin disease — or any skin disease for that matter — because I know how bad it feels to have it and to feel so helpless. I want to share my journey and hope it can make a difference for a lot of you out there. Starting with the cleanse and these simple food groups changed my life. I am aware that everyone is different, our bodies and personalities are all so different, but just remember you have nothing to lose but your red scaly patches and severe itching! By the way, I believe my journey can help anyone with any skin or inflammatory condition, not just psoriasis. So, give it a try. Start slowly if you need to, but do start. Your skin and your health will thank you.

Ps: When you eat healthy food you feel better. You will be cleaner when you start eating greener.

Meditation

I have the strength and desire to get better. This morning I will start with warm lemon water. Sip it slowly and really taste it. (How does it make you feel? Warm, healthy, loving?) I will continue to do it every morning to heal my skin. I am ready to make changes and will start with this.

Next will be food. Baby steps. I will take baby steps to take back control of my health. It feels really good to be the one in control.

When you eat something healthy, sit with it for a moment and think about how well you are taking care of yourself. Be proud of yourself, for every little step you take. Tell yourself how proud you are, how loved you are, and how healthy you already are. Congratulations, you are about to enter a new eating lifestyle and become healthier than you ever imagined!

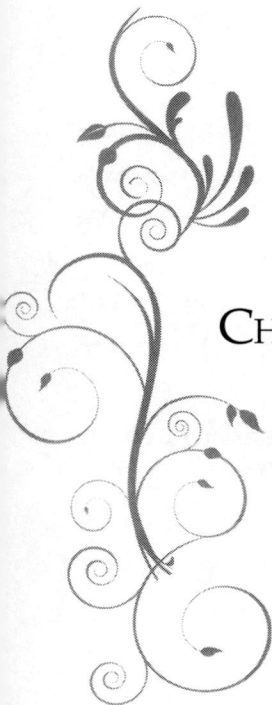

Chapter Eight
Things You Never Thought You Would Do to Your Body

*If you don't take care of this
the most magnificent machine
that you will ever be given...
where are you going to live?*

Karyn Calabrese

When people are asked what the largest organ in your body is, they often forget that it truly is the skin. It seems we never take it as seriously or feel it is as important as the liver, kidneys, or heart. But, the multitude of purposes the skin serves are far-reaching. From your protective cover to sweating when you are too hot to exfoliating to create new skin to regenerating when wounded or burned — the list goes on. And just like all organs of your body, it helps you heal, especially when you have taken the time to detoxify internally first.

When most people think of a healing journey and cleanses, they think of a process that works from the inside out. In Chapter Seven we learned how necessary internal cleansing is for our ultimate health. That said, I'm now going to help you see that what you put on your skin *after* you worked so hard to clean from the inside out is just as crucial to your healing progress.

Beware, because some of the things I talk about in this chapter are not easy to do or to even talk about, but the more you know, the quicker you can heal.

In my particular healing journey, as I worked to become more alkaline starting in the summer of 2012, every day I planned my meals the best I could. When I ate out with friends, I ate as healthily as I could. I drank the teas and followed the cleansing diet. But this was only half of the process. I also took Dead Sea salt baths every week, went for colonics, used coconut oil on my skin instead of my regular lotion, and learned about all the chemicals and toxins — that come from the outside, not just from what we eat — that become trapped inside of us. With a lot of commitment, I started seeing a difference in my skin in a few months.

To help you understand the process, in this chapter, I will be exploring everything from lotions, to colonics, to baths, to the use of clay, to a Squatty Potty; you name it, I share it.

I am going to start with coconut oil because, in the last few years, it has become more widely talked about for all its healing uses. It can be used in literally hundreds of different ways. And if you are one of those people who can't stand shredded coconut or coconut-flavored candies, think again; the real oil has a wonderful flavor, and with all its healing properties, it is worth giving this another try. (One word of advice, get 100 percent virgin coconut oil if possible.) I use it as lotion on my skin as well as keep it as a staple in the kitchen, and I'll talk more about the lotion aspect a bit later.

In the kitchen, I use it in a variety of ways. I heat it to sauté food on the stove, I add it to all my vegan desserts, I add it to my smoothies, and even add a little in my coffee substitutes. The list of benefits is very long, but the main reasons I like to get it in my system every day is that it contains fatty acids that fight inflammation, and its antioxidants are very healing for us skin sufferers. It also prevents all sorts of diseases, including cancer and heart disease, it helps fight overgrowths of bad bacteria, fungus, and viruses, it helps in the digestion process — the list really does go on and on. If you have to choose a "must buy" for your new pantry list, coconut oil should be number one.[24]

A few other items that are now staples in my kitchen — that not only bring some interesting flavor, but help fight inflammation as well — are turmeric, cinnamon, herbs like parsley and mint, ginger, and of course, garlic (which, curiously, is of the lily family).

Let me start with turmeric, a valuable spice that has been getting more attention recently as a healing aid to arthritis and other conditions and diseases. It is an Indian spice that is known to heal. It is anti- everything: oxidant, fungal, viral, bacterial, cancerous — you name it, it's a healer, and you want it in your diet. I sprinkle as much as I can on my veggies while cooking, and I also recently discovered the actual root that I can buy at the health food store, so I started to juice a small piece of it in my green juice here and there. (A word of warning: turmeric stains, especially when in a hot liquid, so cook with caution!)

You can also buy it in capsule form, for those of you who don't cook often, and if you are about to partake in a late

---

24   An excellent website to read up on all things coconut oil is at http://www.draxe.com. The videos there are excellent too. Don't forget to watch the one about psoriasis.

evening of dining and indulging, you can take a few capsules before you go out to help you in the digestion and clearing process.

Cinnamon is another one of those spices that has so many beneficial properties and is gaining momentum as a healing food, especially for diabetes. I'm sure you are all familiar with it, but I'm not talking about the cinnamon and sugar spread we grew up with on our white bread with butter. Although that was one of my favorites as a child, I now use cinnamon as much as I can in my baking, as well as sprinkle it on top of my coffee replacements. It's famous for lowering blood sugar and is a true inflammatory fighter. It's also great in smoothies and can even be used in your tea or with pure cocoa.

As for herbs, the one I use most is fresh parsley. I add a bit to my green juice or chop it up to add to a homemade pot of chicken soup. Parsley has tons of nutrients and vitamins. It contains folic acid, which is one of the critical B vitamins that most of us don't get enough of. Vitamin B keeps our cells healthy and helps prevent diseases such as cancer. It is great to add to smoothies, but be careful how much you add, because it can work as a bowel cleanser and diuretic. If you have edema (swelling), for example, in your body or feet, you can make a parsley tea or take parsley tablets and it will help reduce the water retention. It works differently for each person, so this is one that I recommend you start with smaller amounts and work up. In many restaurants, parsley is served on the way out of the restaurant or even at your table because if you chew on it and spit it out, it freshens your breath from the smell of garlic and other strong herbs.

Mint is another flavor I like because of the minty-fresh taste it gives to my green juice. I have a little plant of it in my kitchen, which my sister-in-law was so sweet to get for me, and I just love it. Mint has so many benefits, but I love it mostly because it helps fight inflammation while giving me fresh breath. Nothing is nicer than a cold glass of water or seltzer in the summer with a sprig of mint, slice of lime, and slice of cucumber poured over ice. Not only is it refreshing but it is also re-hydrating, and this is so important.

Ginger is one of my favorites, and I use this often. I put a small slice each morning in my cup of hot water with lemon. I also juice a small chunk to include in my green juice. I've had it in Asian meals before but haven't attempted to cook with it yet. I also use the dried powder version when baking desserts. Ginger is originally from India. However, there is something called China ginger that is said to be full of nutrients that powerfully help fight inflammation, pain, fatigue, sicknesses such as nausea, and is great to have when you are home sick with a cold or the flu. It is also good to have a ginger tea or even to suck on a piece if your stomach is upset due to nerves or over-indulgence—which is about to happen less and less in your life because the entire goal of this journey is about finding balance!

Garlic is now one of my favorite vegetables. You probably don't see it as a vegetable because you wouldn't eat the entire clove raw, but think of it like an onion. It is known as one of the world's healthiest foods. It adds so much flavor to your dishes, as well as being an excellent source of nutrients such as manganese, vitamin B6, vitamin C, and selenium. It helps lower cholesterol, reduces the risk of heart disease, and its anti-inflammatory properties are said to be amazing! I like to buy the frozen minced chunks from Trader Joe's.[25]

---

25 If buying prepared garlic, you should opt for minced over whole peeled; here's an excellent article on how to get the most benefits from garlic: http://www.enonvalleygarlic.com/about-garlic.html.

You can find a package of them in the frozen section, and when I'm cooking veggies, I pop some out right into the pan. It adds delicious flavor to my meals. I also sometimes buy it fresh, such as when I need to make fresh pickles and the recipe calls for chopped fresh garlic. There are many ways to get it into your food. One favorite is to bake cloves of garlic and smear it on Italian bread—yum! My Italian bread days are over, but I still enjoy soft cloves of it mixed in with my veggies.

Funny story about garlic, though, as most of you know: it does tend to come out of your pores if you eat too much of it. One night I went to this fabulous vegan café with some fellow students from the Institute for Integrative Nutrition. I had this delicious veggie plate covered in soft garlic cloves. They were so good, and I made sure to smear them all over my veggies so I could get the taste in every bite. I came home that night and crawled into bed with Mike after brushing my teeth and washing my face. He woke up to kiss me goodnight and said, "What did you eat tonight? Garlic?" I said yes, and apologized for the smell. (I wasn't really sorry; I really enjoyed that meal!) We fell asleep and in the middle of the night he woke me up to ask me to please not eat that much garlic ever again because he couldn't stand the smell. I guess that's why people eat garlic in meals with each other, because then no one can tell who the smell is coming from. I did feel bad about that because the next morning, he mentioned it again, and no matter how much you brush your teeth, it takes time to dissipate. Let's just say that, when I asked how bad could it be, I got shot one of those dirty looks. Apparently, it was pretty bad. So, sorry Mike! And note to self and readers: don't consume an entire bulb of garlic unless you have a co-conspirator, and don't expect the smell to go away anytime too soon!

There are a ton of other herbs and spices I would highly suggest you explore: sage, rosemary, thyme, dill, basil, cilantro, and oregano (but make sure you go easy on that last one!) I use dill specifically to make fresh pickles. Yup, I now make pickles! Email me and I will be happy to send the recipe to you. Have fun with exploring new spices and find some recipes that use different ones to see which ones you enjoy. These spices will all help you heal your skin.

Now for the items I use directly on my skin. My favorite by far is coconut oil because it's a natural oil that soothes and protects the skin without any chemicals or additives. It dries nicely and is not sticky or tacky as you might think. It has vitamin E and protein, which protects the skin against cracking, prevents premature aging and wrinkling, and keeps the skin healthy and rejuvenated. It has wonderful antioxidant properties and is known to be the most important ingredient in many skin care products today because it doesn't become rancid compared to many other oils. Because of this, it works for a longer time. I love it, and my skin loves it!

I've also tried a few other natural products over the years that are worth mentioning and might help you because you never know what's going to help your special skin. I've heard of these oils and combinations of oils from numerous people, and they've all had success with them:

- **Castor oil**: This anti-inflammatory and anti-oxidant oil has been used for centuries for its health benefits. It also strengthens the immune system, so it's a great remedy for many illnesses and ailments. Dr. Pagano mentions in his book how it has more benefits than people even know about. He has successfully used it for warts, sprains, and strains in athletic injuries. I simply apply a small amount directly on my problem spots when they pop up. It's sticky, so I'll use it only when I know I can wear shorts or a short sleeve shirt, whether I'm home or out. I just don't recommend covering it up with clothing. I wouldn't want them to stick to you or for you to stain them. (By the way, you can find most of these oils in your nearest health food stores, but I order them all on Amazon. Anything to make life easier!)

- **Witch hazel mixed with glycerin**: This anti-inflammatory remedy has healing properties that relieves itch and brings moisture to the skin. Glycerin is a simple sugar alcohol compound. It is colorless, odorless, and sticky, which is why I like to mix it with witch hazel, an astringent, anti-inflammatory compound, produced from the leaves and bark of the witch hazel shrub. Like I said, both can be applied to reduce inflammation on the skin. I have spoken with numerous people with severe Ps who have had fantastic results doing this. I just mix a very small amount (about the size of a quarter) of each together and apply it. Just like with the castor oil, it's still a bit sticky, so try to do this while wearing clothing that doesn't contact the area. You can always apply it, then use Saran Wrap around it before you get dressed. I'm not sure how comfortable that would be all day at work, but I've done it while I slept and it was fine. The evening might be a better solution for you, especially if you have Ps in a more intimate area and, in that case, you might just choose to use a cotton gauze wrap that will let the areas breathe.

- **Hemp seed oil**: This is often used as a moisturizer and has been proven to dramatically decrease skin dryness to alleviate itching and irritation. The antioxidant and anti-inflammatory properties protect against the aging process as well. Hemp seed oil is also a good source of omega-3 and omega-6 fatty acids. I'm sure you are all familiar with hemp seeds. They are a complete protein and may be the most nutritious seed in the world, so eat them up and slather on the oil.

- **Aloe vera**: You probably know that aloe vera is known to heal wounds. It is also known to soothe skin. This clear gel is located inside of the plant and oozes out when you break off a piece. It has several properties that help fight aging, act as a moisturizer, and are effective in treating skin conditions. I use it every summer on my sunburn (because I always get sunburned by accident at least once). According to the Mayo Clinic, it shows some promise in treating more serious and persistent conditions such as eczema, genital herpes, dandruff, psoriasis, canker sores, skin ulcers, and others. Aloe vera is commonly available, but check the label because you want 100 percent aloe vera, not a gel they call aloe vera that has 10 percent aloe and 90 percent alcohol or some other chemical.

- **Peanut oil and almond oil**: These anti-inflammatory and antioxidant oils help promote skin health. These oils are rich in vitamin E, as well as a number of other minerals and vitamins, which helps heal the skin. I follow Dr. Pagano's instructions when I use these: I mix them together, an equal quarter-size amount of each, and massage it onto the problem areas. It helps prevent cracking of the spots or lesions and is great to use especially in the winter when the weather is cold. Dr. Pagano suggests using this mixture above all others when at home since it helps heal the surface cells and it enhances the skin's pliability. Again, don't cover it up with clothing. Not only will you stain your clothes, but they will smell like peanuts. Also, please do not use these if you have a nut allergy.

- **Tea tree oil**: This has helped me heal the Ps in my nails. I'll apply it with a Q-tip into the nails that have lifted a little bit off of the bed due to Ps. I always notice such a difference after a few months. Tea tree oil has too many benefits to list — everything from ringworm to dandruff. I love it because it's known for relieving skin inflammation, which anyone with skin issues can appreciate. It's derived from Australia's tea trees, of which there are over 300 species. Crazy, right? I also love using it as an essential oil in my diffuser to breathe in at night. I love adding it to my Dead Sea salt scrub I make for the shower, which I will discuss below. It smells wonderful. I usually buy this from Trader Joe's as it's cheaper there than at other name-brand stores.

- **Dead Sea salt**: Dead Sea salt baths have shown to drastically improve the skin tissues of many psoriasis sufferers as well as improve blood circulation and eliminate toxins. Visiting the Dead Sea has always been on my to-do list since it's known to be a miraculous healing place to visit. I used to take these baths regularly and absolutely saw a positive difference in my skin. Then I moved to a new apartment with no bathtub and, well, let's just say I look forward to having a bathtub again. In the meantime, I have developed my own Dead Sea salt scrub to use in the shower, which is incredibly soothing and healing. I mix Dead Sea salt with three oils, coconut, vitamin E, and tea tree. These are all excellent ingredients to use on your skin in whichever way works for you. There are tons of recipes for scrubs online, just search away and find one that you want to try. I buy Dead Sea salt online from a company called Midwest Salt Company. The prices are great for a huge twenty-pound bag that will last me for a long time!

- **Calcium bentonite clay**: Something else I do every day for my skin that you might find a bit odd is consume clay. Yes, clay! It's actually 100 percent calcium bentonite clay, and it's known as nature's best-kept secret. Just think about how many toxins we come across every day, whether it's pesticides sprayed on our fruit or scrubbing our house with cleaning products. Most of us breathe in car exhaust every day. A lot of people also consume a ton of processed food, which are full of chemicals and preservatives.

Whether you drink or eat clay, or even take it as a supplement, it acts as a magnet while moving through your body, attracting and removing all of the toxins, heavy metals, foreign substances, and impurities from the gut, skin, and mouth as it passes through you. Clay has negatively charged electrons and most toxins and heavy metals have positively charged electrons, so this allows the two to bind together easily while the toxin removal process happens. I drink a small capful each morning and night. It doesn't really taste like anything, but does leave your mouth dry, so have some water ready to drink afterward. Its primary functions are to alkalize the body, relieve digestive issues, allow cells to receive more oxygen, and boost immunity. Below is a list of other ways it helps us internally. I guarantee you'll read this and want to start consuming clay as soon as possible! Benefits of calcium bentonite clay:

o Removes heavy metals
o Rids the body of yeast and candida
o Helps reduce gas and bloating
o Aids recovery from chemotherapy and radiation
o Eliminates internal parasites
o Increases absorption of vitamins and nutrients
o Detoxifies the liver
o Heals ulcers and acid reflux
o Helps with Crohn's disease and colitis
o Boosts the immune system
o Stops vomiting and diarrhea
o Gets rid of hangovers
o Stops food poisoning
o Alkalizes the body
o Helps with morning sickness

You can also use clay externally. I often apply it on a cotton ball and rub it directly on my stubborn Ps spots, but you can also use it for any insect bites, cuts, skin itching, burns, rashes, or other skin conditions. It is known to be very calming for skin itching for us Ps sufferers. I buy a product that is more of a liquid to drink directly out of the bottle, but if you choose to buy it in a thicker form, you can mix it with water before applying to your skin. You would apply it, let it sit for a while until it dries and then wash it off. You should talk to the company representative about how to use it, but there are also directions on the container as well as online. I buy a brand called Cleansing Concepts. It's a company I know and trust. You can order directly from them online or, if you're in the New York area, from one of their three stores here (two in Long Island and one in Brooklyn). From wherever you get your clay, beware; there are clays out there that can be acidic and contaminated. So, do your research, go with a recommendation, or simply ask the company for proof purity and its pH levels.

And now for something no one wants to talk about, but I need to share: colon hydrotherapy. I know, just the word alone has sent you to the end of this book and out the door. "Ain't no way I'm going there!" I hear you. But hang on. There are different levels and components of this process, and when something works, it's amazing how far we will go to feel good, and this does work.

Also known as colonics, this is not for everyone. If you have suffered from any form of irritable bowel syndrome, rectal bleeding from any unhealed lesions, Crohn's, or unhealed unremoved polyps, then this is most likely not for you at the moment. I admit I was a bit wary—well, more than a bit—when I first read about it in Dr. Pagano's book. Colonics is a process where toxins get flushed from your intestinal tract by injecting water into the colon via tubes in your rectum. The water is filtered, warm, and is slowly released into the colon, causing your colon muscles to contract and push everything back out through the hose. The process lasts anywhere between thirty to forty-five minutes and, not to put it too indelicately, you will be shocked at the amount of fecal matter that comes out.

Fecal matter accumulates and hardens in the colon, and this buildup negatively affects our health. It can prevent the absorption of water and nutrients, lead to constipation, allow harmful colon bacteria and yeast to grow, and cause stagnant toxins to be absorbed into the bloodstream through the colon wall. Today's standard Western diet—with a lack of fiber, excess sugar, and high in red meat—is believed to contribute to the problem. While our bodies are well equipped to cleanse themselves and know what to do, cleansing through the use of colonics made such sense to me.

I committed to trying every method of healing that Dr. Pagano suggested, so the first thing I did was ask around. I thought of my friends who would be open to this type of conversation and, sure enough, I got two recommendations for the same practitioner, Diane Paxton.[26] From my very first visit with her, I felt safe! That's my biggest piece of advice when it comes to trying a colonic: get a recommendation.

I started going to Diane for colonics five years ago and, over the years, she has become my regular practitioner whom I go to for Nutritional Response Testing (NRT) and all my whole food supplements. (I'll explain more about NRT later.) Getting a colonic can be a bit uncomfortable. As the water slowly fills your intestines, you feel cramping, and it feels very relieving to finally release that water and all that comes

---

26   Diane Paxton is with Inner Fire Integrative Health Services located in Brooklyn, NY.

out with it. This process is repeated the entire time, in and out. The first time you go will probably be the worst, not so much because of the cramping but because you don't know what to expect. Your mind is playing games with you, especially knowing someone is going to be putting a tube up your behind! The process is very private and personal, but I don't find it uncomfortable when it's administered by someone nurturing. That's why it's incredibly important in my opinion to go to someone recommended.

When my practitioner moved and was no longer nearby, I started going to a wellness center called Cleansing Concepts. This center runs very differently because you are alone in the room and administer the colonic yourself. The water flow is regulated, and you can call an attendant or stop the water anytime. They also check on you every ten minutes. I feel very safe there, as well, and it's now more convenient for me because it's closer to my home. So, do your research and know you have options. I can completely understand if people are just not open to it. Like I said, it's not for everyone. I wanted to include it here because it is a part of my healing regimen, and for those of you who might be open to it, I wanted to give you an inside look.

What keeps me going there regularly is how good I feel afterward. It leaves me feeling — well, cleaned out...light, empty, and, mentally, knowing I'm doing everything I can to heal myself. That's why I don't mind the uncomfortable feeling that comes with it. I've even kind of started to enjoy it; not the process, mind you, but the results and how I feel afterward.

〜

If I got the best of you by just mentioning the word colonics, don't worry, I have a different, pain-free, invasive-free treatment that really works; but keep an open mind because you would think that the days of *Star Trek* have arrived when you learn more about it. It's called Nutrition Response Testing (NRT). I have continued this as a main part of my health routine. I started NRT two years ago. It was initially a twelve-week program, and now I go every few months. I must say, NRT is unlike anything I've ever experienced, and I find it very hard to explain. When I talk about it, it sounds very "woo-woo" and people tend to look at me a little funny.

NRT is a way of analyzing the body to determine where you have nutritional deficiencies that may be causing any illness or poor health you are experiencing. The practitioner will test your neurological reflexes by extending one arm with one hand while contacting a specific reflex area with the other hand. If the tested reflex is stressed, your nervous system will respond by reducing energy to your extended arm, causing it to weaken and drop. Though it may not sound so, it's actually very scientific. Dr. Mark Goldhirsch, a chiropractor, explains it well:

> The analysis tests the body's neurological reflexes and acupuncture points. The neurological reflexes are derived from the part of the nervous system whose job it is to regulate the functions of each and every organ. The acupuncture points are selected from the ancient Chinese system of acupuncture which is thousands of years old. Nutrition Response Testing is a study of how the different points on the surface of the body relate to the state of health and to the flow of energy in each and every organ and function of the body. Interestingly, since the human anatomy has not changed significantly

in thousands of years, the utilization of these reflex-es and specific points have become extremely use-ful in my practice because they are so accurate. Each Nutrition Response Testing reflex represents a specific organ, tissue, or function, and indicates the effect that energy, or the lack of energy, is having on the body. By testing the Nutrition Response Testing reflexes, we have a system of monitoring your body at each visit that has proven to be extremely accurate clinically and that helps us identify exactly what the body needs and how well we are meeting that need.[27]

Just to give you a small example, my practitioner had me raise my right arm straight out in front of me. I was able to resist her pressure pushing down on my right arm. Then she put the tiniest amount of sugar granules in my left hand. Not only could I not resist her, but my arm came down so fast, it had zero strength. I know sugar is toxic to our bodies, but this one small test movement showed me exactly how detrimental it is in my body! It was fascinating.

After the testing is complete and the cause is determined, the practitioner will design a program using nutrition and whole food supplements to help you heal. Vitamin deficien-cies can lead to a wide range of health issues, so it's crucial to take the right ones. After my first test, my practitioner found heavy metals and fungus in my body, which we eliminated over time by cleaning up my diet and testing which supple-ments worked best for me. I had brought her all of my current supplements that I had always bought over the years from a convenient vitamin store.

---

27   http://drmarkg.com/nutrition/nutrition-response-testing.html.

Those included fish oil, a multivitamin, and vitamin D. To my surprise, they tested negative to having any effect on my body, and I'm sure that was because they were manufactured synthetically with chemicals and did not come straight from their natural sources. Vitamins should be made directly from the plant containing the vitamin, not produced in a lab. Many vitamin and mineral supplements are developed this way, and they are made to imitate the way natural, real vitamins perform in our bodies. Many experts believe we are destroying our health this way. It reminds me of processed foods and GMOs: now we know that if it's not real, not to put it in our bodies, right? Supplements are a wonderful way to get the vitamins the body needs to heal and prevent disease. The Organic Consumer's Organization explains the importance of taking supplements well:

In today's world, it's virtually impossible to do well without nutritional supplements. Supplementation often presents the only practical means to grant an adequate intake of nutrients. Due to soil depletion, industrial food processing, storage conditions and often low accessibility to fresh nutrient-dense food, it becomes imperative to supplement our diet with vitamins and other essential nutrients which are missing in our food. And the people who need supplementation most, are those under an increased oxidative stress including people routinely engaged in intense physical training, people with immune-deficiency diseases, and the elderly. Antioxidant nutrients have shown to help lower the metabolic stress caused by exercise or disease and thus protect cells and tissues from oxidative damage.[28]

---

28   https://www.organicconsumers.org/news/vitamin-poisoning-are-we-destroying-our-health-hi-potency-synthetic-vitamins.

The only other thing I want to stress about vitamins is that they are not all created alike. Try to purchase a brand from an actual health food store versus a Walmart, because they have done their research and only stock brands that keep their vitality. Many vitamins sold on the market no longer have any vitality at all, so you are wasting your money and your energy swallowing them.

Our diets and lifestyle choices are constantly changing the needs of our bodies, too. The supplements I started out taking in this program are not the ones I take today. When I see my health practitioner every few months, she might add or take away something to keep me balanced, all depending on what is going on in me at that time. My daily vitamins tend to be probiotics, a multi-vitamin, and fish oil. I used to buy random brands of fish oil from a local pharmacy, not ever thinking about how they were developed. All I ever did was go out of my way to avoid the ones that made me taste the fishy flavor when burping. Since then, I've found a good quality one (without the burps!) They're from Nordic Naturals, and my body loves them. The benefits of fish oil encompass everything from reducing joint pain and cardiovascular disease to improving skin and enhancing mental health. It's worth exploring them more.

If you are open to trying NRT, I would highly recommend it as it has become a staple in my healing practice and helps me tremendously (and it is pain-free!) You could also see your MD to get your blood work done to figure out what they suggest your body needs. If there is a health food store near you, pop in and check out all of the various brands of natural vitamins it offers. Talk to the staff about which they suggest you try, then see what the internet says about it. Do your research and find a company that you believe in and feel is a safe option for you.

And now, it's time to talk about the Squatty Potty. Yes, you read that correctly, and I bet you have already guessed, we are now going to talk about our poop!

Dr. Oz is the one who has pushed the movement of it being okay to discuss our poop, but once you get the hang of it, the easier it becomes. My husband jokes about buying me a t-shirt that says, "I pooped today," because, apparently, I like talking about poop. It is something that gets easier once you get the hang of analyzing it, and once you start looking at it, you will see it is a beautiful indication of your health. Mike says he hates when I talk about it, but I think somewhere deep down he finds it humorous.

So, back to the Squatty Potty. I was first introduced to the Squatty Potty when I had my first colonic and since then I've been hooked. Using a bathroom without one just isn't the same. Whenever new friends come over and use the bathroom, they come out asking, "What is that thing under your toilet?" It happens nearly every time. And every time I say, proudly, "It's a Squatty Potty, and it's life-changing!"

The Squatty Potty is like a small curvy step stool that slides to fit perfectly under your toilet so it can be tucked away when you're not using it. When it's time to poop, you just pull it out and prop your feet up on it. What this does is raise your knees higher than your hips, which helps loosen up your body, aligns your bowels properly, and makes elimination much easier and faster. Our bodies were designed to squat when defecating, which relaxes the muscle around the colon and allows the colon to open up and empty without any blockage. With our modern-day toilets having us sitting down, that muscle is only partially relaxed and some toxic waste could get blocked. That buildup of toxic waste in the colon could end up causing all sorts of health issues, including colon cancer. This simple tool could help prevent hemorrhoids, constipation, straining, bloating, colon cancer, IBS, hernias, and diverticulosis. I must say, I've become quite the Squatty Potty enthusiast. I used to be very secretive about all things excreted because I was embarrassed, but now I rave about it because it has changed my life.

They are shockingly inexpensive, running at only $25 for a basic plastic one, and can be ordered from Amazon or directly from the company that makes them at squattypotty.com. I have to tell you, it has become my signature gift to friends who get pregnant or complain to me about their pooping issues. They always love it, and it's a funny surprise!

Well, I won't torture you anymore on the crazy things that help you heal, and I've purposely kept the chapter short because I know this may all be new to you. Let me end again on the simple fact that there are so many things we can lovingly do working from the outside in, things that compliment your internal cleanse and get you to ultimate healing and health more quickly, so just try to have an open mind!

⬱

Ps: Be open-minded and experiment. By trying new things, you may happen upon something that works more quickly and is better than you would have ever guessed. Your body will thank and love you for it!

Meditation

Stop what you're doing right now. Yes, stop reading. Look at a part of your body that brings you negative thoughts and repeat the following: I am committed to your healing. I am ready to feel confident about you. Show me the way to what will help you and I promise to be open to whatever that may be. You are now my priority. It's time for us to feel happy together. I love you and am ready, so show me the way.

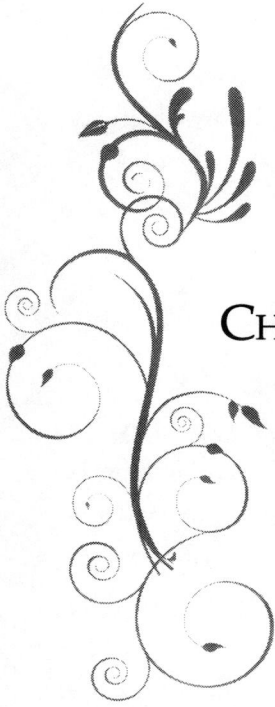

CHAPTER NINE
Emotional Triggers: Our Bodies Really Do Talk to Us

There is deep wisdom in our flesh, if we can only come to our senses and feel it.

Elizabeth A. Behnke

One of the most amazing things about human beings is that we are so much more than bones wrapped in a layer of skin or organs that function independently of each other. We are complex beings that have physical components that need to work with each other, emotional reactions that are not so easily defined, and spiritual dimensions that are so diverse and personal it would take another book to address. Each one of these areas—mind, body, and spirit—make up a human, and each human is completely different. If you think about that concept itself, it is overwhelming. Imagine trying to think of a way to help all psoriasis sufferers or all people who suffer from certain diseases. It is a daunting task. So, sometimes the best way to help people is to share what you have learned and let others pick and choose what works for them. I know my story and know how I learned what works for me. I'm also painfully aware that it might not always work for others. There is no magic sauce. One thing that I have learned that works is never to coach people to do what I do, but to help guide them to figure out what works for them.

In this chapter, I am going to address what I have found to be the most common emotional triggers that individuals with skin disorders suffer from, because I think there is little that is dermatologically superficial about this disorder. Being aware of mind, body, and spirit is what will move you to health so much more quickly. I will explore this in sections related to topics such as negative thinking, anger, shame, and insecurity, and then provide some ideas and ways to manifest change through actually changing your perception and behavior, and moving in a positive direction.

I am going to start with an issue we all struggle with on a daily basis: self-control. You know and I know that this is not just a behavior, it is an emotional reaction to a choice or an idea long before it becomes a positive or negative action. If we could all just simply do what we are supposed to—eat the healthiest foods, meditate, exercise, stay away from toxins of all kinds, laugh, enjoy our work, and be happy—we would all have exercised perfect self-control, and we would all most likely be healthy. But, life just does not work that way, and self-control is no easy issue. I want to begin by sharing some issues I have had with self-control, which is something I need to pay attention to every single day, many times during the day, and my guess is you do too.

I wrote in journals on and off throughout the years, but it wasn't until I started acting classes at thirty years old that I learned about a book called *The Artist's Way*, by Julia Cameron.[29] Her book changed my world, and I recommend you all read it and follow the writing exercises. Curiously, seven years later, Julia ended up being my teacher for a week at the Institute for Integrative Nutrition, at which point I was reminded to pick up the book again. Her book introduces you to doing what she calls morning pages, where you wake up and write down anything that comes to mind. It could be your to-do list for the day or a simple thought about something that happened at work — it doesn't matter. You just get every single thought you have out on paper. The point of this is to empty your mind as much as possible so you can experience more creativity in your life. She believes we all have creativity and, by doing this exercise every day, we allow it to come through once we get our cacophony of thoughts out of the way. This is a beautiful way to journal.

However you do it, journaling will help you grow and develop. It allows you to see what you've written and gain so much insight into your life. I find it releases stress too. All I know is, when I did the Artist's Way exercise, my life shifted in a very subtle way that is hard to explain. My acting was more truthful, my communication was better, and my self-esteem improved. I believe it affects us in very subconscious ways.

I want to share some notes that popped out at me when I was re-reading my journal to come up with some ideas for this book. Here is an entry:

---

29   Yes, I keep a journal and recommend you do too; it is the most cleansing and awakening thing you can do because when you read it down the road you will smile at the progress you made. You will realize new things as they pop out at you. Things so obvious now but you might not have ever recognized them before. It's amazing what you see years later after you have put it down for a while!

I feel like I'm at a plateau. I don't think it's food at this point; I think it's mental. I want so badly not to think about my Ps for one minute or one entire day. It feels like it runs my life, not me running my life. I remember feeling in such control years back. I remember feeling so empowered learning I was in control. I could heal myself, and my Ps had no say in the matter. What happened? When did I lose control? I feel helpless at this moment and trust me it's the last thing I want to write about, but you, Universe, and anyone that reads this, are on this journey with me now, so you're on this emotional roller coaster with me. I have spots popping up on my legs and scalp now. I'm feeling very discouraged lately. I've been so focused working hard for four months now on my eating, and it started looking amazing at one point. But then it came back on one elbow and not the other. Could this have to do with the steroid from my bursitis draining two times? (*I was struggling with that as well at the time I wrote this.*) It doesn't make sense ... I just feel over this whole diet. I feel done focusing on every piece of food I put in my mouth. I want to live my life and enjoy it. I'm feeling helpless and out of control. It sucks! I am thinking a lot of it may be mental. Mike thinks so. He thinks I need to not pay so much attention to it. That makes sense because like attracts like and I believe in the law of attraction. You get what you expect, and I expect to see Ps on my body because I don't know anything else. But, how do I not pay attention to it when I see it every day? I'm feeling a bit depressed about it.

This journal entry hit me because I know absolutely everyone who reads this has experienced these types of emotions at one point or another. Depression and anger are the very first emotions that come to mind when disease is present, and both these emotions need to be dealt with, but other ones include shame, insecurity, fear, guilt, helplessness, and sadness. I encourage you, from this point forward, whether it is with a therapist, a good friend, a support group, a doctor, a guru, or your journal, you must find the time to acknowledge and come to terms with these feelings. The acceptance of our emotions is something I have worked on only recently in my life and is still something I work on daily. My advice to people for years was always "just feel your feelings, that's all you can do" when it came to a loss, disappointment, pain, etc., but I had a very hard time taking my own advice and I believe all of that emotional repression contributed to my Ps. It has to come out somehow or somewhere doesn't it?

To make the process of release easier to follow, I have broken down the categories so you can come back and read them on days when one emotion seems to be overriding others.

Depression

Everyone struggles with depression and down days now and then, and when you are dealing with a chronic illness, it does make it harder to fight through, because your mind is in constant overdrive trying to deal with and process what is happening and what you need to do. So, I have to say, no matter what, expect some down days. They are going to happen to all of us.

This condition, in particular, has a way of creeping up on you when you least expect it, and it will make you feel like you are the one who is not in control. It's so easy to feel down when your skin is flared up with any condition. Let's face it, you feel ugly — and I don't know about you, but I've had my days where I've doubted if anyone out there was ever going to love me in a romantic way because of it. I've also doubted my own worth because of it in many different situations. I remember getting a flare-up on my leg once when shooting an indie horror flick, where most of the film took place hiking in the woods. Thankfully, we had our choice of wardrobe. But, as such, I was the only female who wore pants — and boy, did I feel less than perfect. I wanted so badly to be like the other girls, have my legs showing in a dress or shorts, and have to be zero percent self-conscious about it in that aspect. It was hot, too. Nothing like wearing pants during long, hot days on set. I was very down about it and didn't know at that point how to love myself enough to relieve some of the pain. I just wasn't my happy self, and that feeling of being down and not having any control was debilitating.

Something I have learned now is that, if I feel down, even to the point of tears, I allow myself to let out a good cry. I mentioned earlier that I had days where I would sit on the toilet or the floor and just cry my eyes out screaming, "Why me?" I must say, just letting it out and releasing that emotion was what I needed at that moment. So, when you're down, try to have a good strong release, and then have a loving chat with yourself. If that doesn't help you even a little, consider letting yourself just be and see if the next day is better. Crying helps release many blocked emotions and resistance. Just know, when you are crying you are releasing toxins your body needs to release to make you healthier, so cry until you can't cry anymore. Crying in therapy sessions or with friends is something that should be encouraged to get it all out. Don't try to hold it in. And if you are a man, forget the saying that real men don't cry. Real men do and should cry, so try it out and don't feel bad. No matter what you do, make sure you are in a safe environment for such a release because there are still a lot of people out there who might judge you for this. Release what you can; there is a good chance that tomorrow will be a better day.

Anger

One day, again while journaling, I came up with this idea: what if this skin disease is from all my anger built up inside of me? What if it never had anything to do with what I ate? What if I created it? When I looked back at some of my journals while writing this book, I came across quite a few that were so full of anger. I was probably the angriest when I was twenty-one and with my friends on spring break. I was in Cancun in my bathing suit with my hot girlfriends, who were so confident, while I was pissed. *Why in the world did the universe pick this moment in time to ruin my life?* I thought. I also liked this guy — who took one look at my legs and looked grossed out while asking what the spots were. Ugh!

That was probably around the time I started believing that no man would ever want to date me if he knew I had Ps. I think it was during that trip that I had a million such negative thoughts. I was angry, as if someone or something was conspiring against me. It just felt like the absolute worst time in my life to cover my legs and, most of all, I was young and jealous of my friends whose biggest issues were, basically, what to wear. That's not totally true, my friend Katie got her tooth broken by a beer bottle. (Okay, so, maybe we assume we have it the worst!)

I also remember feeling anger more recently when I was eating well and doing everything that had healed me at the beginning of my journey, yet this spot on my leg was being very stubborn and would not go away. Oh boy, was I mad! My poor husband has witnessed many episodes of me pacing through the apartment saying, "But I just don't get it? I don't understand! I'm doing everything right!"

That's when I would find myself thinking, *Maybe it was that one thing I ate,* or *Maybe it's because I didn't eat a lot of greens last week!* That's where Mike would come in and say, "Um, I'm pretty sure it's the stress of juggling a million things on your plate right now." And I'd be blown away that he was able to figure it out before me.

When you feel angry, just feel it until eventually it subsides, because it will. I wish I would have done that more: just accept the anger when I did feel it, and not repress it or avoid it or pretend it didn't exist. Another tool is only to allow yourself to sit with anger, fear, or rejection for so many minutes and then force yourself to do something positive or that you enjoy. Often, just moving into a different space or tricking your mind to be busy on another topic, and praising the good things, will help you start to feel a release. I am not asking you to repress. You acknowledge first, see if you can learn anything from the response, and then you try to release it by replacing the angry thoughts with positive ones.

Shame

Interestingly, when I think about my emotions through the years, I'd say of all of them, this was the one I've struggled

with the most. I felt shamed by my Ps. It had this way of making me feel humiliated which was so painful. When people
feel this way, they usually lower their heads or avoid eye contact, or you see it in the way they hold their posture. For me,
it was covering my body in clothing. I bet it's that way for a
lot of people struggling with a lot of different things such as
weight, skin conditions, and who-knows-what.

Shame is the one emotion that was with me most of the
time. The feelings of sadness and anger would subside, but
not the shame. I've carried shame around with me for sixteen
years, like a heavy weight on my back, like we're old friends
(that hate each other!). I still have a small burst of it if I have
a flare-up. Now, though, I simply have a loving conversation
with myself and don't drag it around with me like I used to.
I know better. It's a wasted emotion, to me. I wasted so many
moments in my life feeling that way when I could have focused on feeling more love for myself.

I can't talk about one specific story here because I honestly
was never without shame all those years. What I can share is
this: when my Ps healed, and I walked around feeling more
confident, I realized the shameful feeling had lifted — and the
words to describe that are endless. The main word I think of is
freeing. It seriously felt like someone had let me out of jail. But
when my Ps returned, that familiar feeling of shame rushed
back in like nobody's business. Now, though, I am aware of
two things: I know what it feels like to not carry that feeling
around with me, and know that I am the one in control of
my thoughts and healing. Boom! These are such important
things you need to know about shame. My journey has taken
me on a search of the question: How do I love myself when I
look at something on my body with such hatred? I have realized, little by little, that this is the answer. The only thing that

healed my shameful thoughts were loving ones! Please, whatever you do, write that down and start being more loving to yourself right now.

Insecurity

I think we can all relate to this emotion, especially when it comes to our bodies. They are never perfect enough are they? Whether it's insecurity about your weight, shape, size, hair, nose, skin, etc., we all have them. I think my most insecure moment with Ps was sometime in my thirties. I was getting intimate with a man and remember him being very touchy-feely, trying to touch me. Meanwhile, I was trying to move so that he wouldn't feel my elbows. I know what you're thinking: *She's so insecure, and this is really what the man is after?* Yes. Yes, I was worried about my elbows! Because, at that time, I didn't accept my skin condition. I resisted it as much as I could. I was scared. I was scared he would feel the roughness and, worse, would stop kissing me to ask me what the hell was on my elbows. Who wants that question in the midst of fooling around? And now I know that, even if he had asked me what it was, it didn't mean he would be so turned off he would stop what he was doing and leave. But, back then, I was plain old scared of what men (anyone!) would think. I was so disgusted by it that I just assumed they would be too.

Some of you may think I was crazy for feeling so scared about something I had no control over, but I know some of you will hear my pain and relate to it. For example, I received an email recently from a man in India who is convinced his wife left him because of his Ps. He said he is covered all over his body, and the flakes are everywhere — on the bed, couch, carpet, etc.—and that his wife couldn't take it anymore. She cheated on him and then left him. He blames it on his Ps. Although I feel it might not all be because of his Ps, it doesn't mean that I don't feel his pain. If I were in his shoes, I would probably feel the same way. Fortunately, he's now starting to heal his body slowly and trying to take control of his disease so he can meet someone else again in the future. I think that what all these emotions do have in common is the need for self-love, even when you are not feeling it. If you are feeling insecure, do something that will help lift some of that emotion. For me, I like to go for a manicure and pedicure; it makes me feel pretty (at least my fingers and toes). Pick a part of your body that you feel good about and focus on that. You will find one, I promise. There are parts of everyone that are just beautiful.

Fear

Next to shame, this is another emotion that I used to carry around with me a lot of the time. I've always feared judgment. I've been scared about what people would think because my thoughts about my Ps have been so cruel. It's called projecting. I think that coming out of the closet about my Ps to others has been a huge step away from fear. What's the worst thing that could happen? Will you not get that job because your potential employer sees your skin covered in red, flaky, patches? Will you not get a date? Will people stare at you?

For me, I mostly feared others thinking something was wrong with me, as though I were a leper and they would fear catching it. With men, I feared they wouldn't be attracted to me, let alone date me. With my acting career, I feared being fired if I couldn't wear shorts or a t-shirt. This was all in my head because, only now, do I see the way my ego was working its evil ways. None of these things even happened to me! I dated a lot, and people wanted to be my friend because they loved who I am, and I even acted in a lot of films without any issues.

So, who is making sure that fear pops up when it's completely unnecessary? My ego! There are only two kinds of fear: real fear and psychological fear. I love and appreciate real fear. I want my body's nervous system to freak out and warn me if I'm about to be attacked. But psychological fear is unhelpful and detrimental to people who want to live a happy and fulfilling life. I still feel fear all the time, but now I stop dead in my tracks, stare it down, and place it by the door and say, "Thanks so much, fear, I appreciate you trying to help me out, but I've got this! Buh-bye!" I hope you start doing the same. Don't accept it and let it run your life—fight back and take control of what you are meant to do here: be joyful!

Helplessness

This feeling is the absolute *worst!* When you feel like you have zero control over any emotions or conditions in your life, it's just the worst feeling. You feel like you're not the one living your life. Recently, I was eating very clean, was back on my alkaline wagon after a slight fall off of it, and after four months I found myself feeling helpless. I was confused and sad and felt this lack of control that doesn't feel good. I know eating clean whole foods heals, so why was the Ps still there after four months? I saw some healing in certain spots, but other spots were popping up, and I couldn't for the life of me figure out why.

This is where my primary food — which we are taught in our school means relationships, career, money, exercise, stress, spiritual practice — came in. My primary food was out of balance, not my food. If any of these categories are out of balance, food will not fix it. That's one thing I learned in school that I will always be grateful for. It was life-changing, learning that. It seems so simple, right? But why, then, are so many people suffering from all sorts of diseases out there?

Once I was so obviously reminded by my hubby that I was under a lot of stress at that time, I was able to take a step back and figure out ways to relieve some of that; once I did that, I started healing! De-stressing myself and eating clean did the trick, but I couldn't have healed without both. I urge you to take a good, long look at your primary life and see where you may have any imbalances you can work on.

Sadness

Sadness, like depression, can make you not want to get out of bed in the morning. As I've mentioned, I have a very naturally upbeat, positive, happy personality, and don't feel good when I'm feeling any other emotion. It just feels off and not good. I enjoy feeling lit up and excited and joyful, and when I find myself around people who are sad or down in some way, I can't help but want to fix them so they can look at things differently and be happier.

When I feel sad, it feels so wrong to me and sometimes I just can't fix myself. Sometimes it takes a bit of time, maybe a few hours or a few days to get back to my normal self. I always do return to my natural state of happy, but in those moments, feeling sad outright sucks! I notice what works for me is staying busy during those times. It's when I make the most plans with friends who are in a happy, positive place. Sometimes, you may not be in the mood to be around others, but you can keep busy in other ways, such as going for a walk, going to the park and reading a book, going to the beach and riding a bike, running errands, cleaning your house, cooking a new recipe, journaling, etc. Do something besides watching TV and trying to numb the pain, unless you pick a humorous and loving movie to watch that will pull you out of your mind and get you into a happy state of being. But afterward, do something a little more active.

I have a friend who works for someone who is ill. She organizes her paperwork and her life and even walks her dog. The woman wanted to hire someone like my friend because she was so happy, bubbly, and positive, always looking at the glass half full. It was important for her to be around someone with her happy personality type because she gets sad at times about her illness and needs that energy around her. I think she's one smart woman, who knows what her soul is craving! So, if you feel sad, keep busy. My favorite thing to do is go for brunch with friends. It always makes me feel so good to be around loving people I care about and to eat healthy, yummy food.

🐚

The biggest lesson I can teach you about emotions is that we all experience them, and just like being prepared with an arsenal of healthy food, prepare yourself with an arsenal of ways to acknowledge the feelings but then move through them.

Like you, I have gone through and still go through all of these emotions. They pop up from time to time, but I can see them now in a different way, like I'm an observer of them. I still feel them, but I don't allow myself to get lost in them like I used to. I hope this encourages you to do the same.

✑

Now, once you have started to make friends with the fact that you will experience all of the above emotions, I would like to teach you some more steps to handling behaviors that technically start from an emotional response and then have the opportunity to take a turn for the worse or a turn for the better, depending on how you control them. Imagine: you may have never realized it, but you do have power over how you allow emotions to control and trigger you!

Willpower/Self-Control

When I first started my journey, I had a ton of willpower because I was *so, so* sick of feeling crappy because of my Ps that I got to a place where I would do *anything* to heal it. I know a lot of people suffering out there who feel the same way. They have 100 percent self-control right now; they are eating the cleanest foods and are feeling great! I also know a lot of people suffering out there who just can't help but feel like it's just too hard to eat this way all the time, and find themselves veering off to have a cup of coffee, a donut, or a cheeseburger.

Then, I see those people who have total self-control in other areas but have a hard time maintaining the diet and lifestyle. We are all so differently wired and handle life in ways that are comfortable to us individually. I struggle with not having hot wings! They are my most favorite food. In the beginning, they were one of the things I missed the most besides coffee. I still struggle with self-control to this day. I hear you.

You may be like me, where it felt easy to me in the beginning because I was super motivated. I think we all feel that way. It's like starting a diet to lose weight after the new year. It's easy because we are all gung-ho, really serious this time, blah, blah, blah. Then we fall off the wagon. The difference here is that this isn't a diet. This is a lifestyle change that our bodies need to feel their best and to operate their best, and once you get in the habit of organizing it, shopping differently, eating differently, thinking differently, it will eventually become your new habit and lifestyle.

Once I started eating healthy, I felt so amazing that I never wanted to go back. I never wanted even to put a potato chip in my mouth. Fast forward through the years to me eating a chip at a barbecue party here and there. Deep down, I don't want that in my body, but my stomach and brain want to taste it even if there are negative consequences.

It's very natural to fall off the wagon, so accept that you *will*. Accept it right now. I think the key to enjoying ourselves on this food journey and in this life is that when we fall off, we say, "Oops, I fell off, let me get back on" without all of the guilt and nasty thoughts about how much we suck. What good does any of that do and, also, are any of those thoughts loving? Focus on self-love here. What is self-love in this situation? Is it to beat yourself up and tell yourself you are not good enough? Or is it to acknowledge that you lost a bit of self-control, and you will add some spinach to that smoothie you're about to have to make up for it?

I was the worst with beating myself up these past few years. We all have our personal standards, and guilt comes rushing in when you know you've compromised them. It's a terrible feeling, and it can paralyze us. The guilt that I carried around with me was heavy, especially as I started to do this work as a health coach. Can you even imagine the thoughts that would go through my mind while I was launching my business? How could I teach people to how to eat to heal their skin when I eat whatever I want 10 percent of the time?

I was at dinner with my mother-in-law recently and decided to enjoy a glass of wine. I had a small spot of Ps on my leg I was working on healing, so should I feel guilty about having that glass of wine? I was at a baby shower a few weekends ago and decided to enjoy a piece of cake, so should I feel guilty? As I write this, I'm still working on healing my leg and thoughts are popping in to say, "Hypocrite!" I look at that thought and say to myself, "Who's telling me that?" Once I ask that question, I am reminded of the ego, the little dark cloud that lurks and tries to ruin our success. I'm eating so healthy 90 percent of the time that when I eat that piece of cake, I should enjoy it immensely without any added emotions — just joy!

I love the journey I'm on because if I weren't going through the same struggles as you, I'd never be able to help you. My message here is to accept where you're at. If you fall off the wagon, which you will often on this journey, just pick up that hat, dust it off, and get back on while reminding yourself how human you are. Again, this all boils down to self-love. I love myself, so I'm not going to allow guilt to force me to be something I'm not — perfect. You will find that that release alone will start to open up room for willpower and self-control to return.

Plateauing

I want to start this section with a blurb from my journal so you can see what I have been through:

I've plateaued! It doesn't feel very good; I feel nothing but stuck. I've been eating mostly alkaline for almost five months now — or I thought I've been eating
mostly alkaline. I somehow strayed from the 80/20
percent alkaline/acidic ratio. For some crazy reason,
I've thought as long as I stay away from white flour,
red meat, and processed foods, I can eat all the brown
rice and chicken that I want! Yeah? No! It's interesting what's happening right now; I have one elbow
that is 90 percent cleared and one that isn't looking so
good! On top of that, when I started writing this book
I didn't have any Ps on my legs, and now I have little
spots here and there, just enough for me to feel self-
conscious and just in time for spring and summer! I'm
feeling bad about this; I just feel like screaming out to
the universe "Why me?"

I've struggled with this most of my life, so there's a huge
part of me that wonders what life must be like to live without
it and how lovely that must be! Then there's another part of
me that wonders what my life would be like without it because it has taught me so much! Strange and unimaginable.

Plateauing is tough! It's outright frustrating. You heal,
you see the progress, you're motivated and then, boom, nothing continues to happen. You feel stuck and may even feel
encouraged to eat even cleaner and stricter, which only brings
on more anger and helplessness if the spots don't clear up
right away. It's a vicious cycle of emotions that plateauing
can bring on. I know, I've plateaued, and it was then I realized I had to look at my primary food to see what changes
I could make to lessen my stress. I also realized that I was

eating a lot more animal protein than veggies. Normally, my veggie intake far outweighed my animal protein intake, but during that time I was busy and allowed myself to get lazy in the kitchen, which means I prepared fewer veggies. Take a look at the alkaline vs. acidic chart I provided in Chapter Four and see if your acidic intake outweighs your alkaline intake. You'll be surprised! And, like I said, take a good long look at your primary food; are you feeling stress at work or are you going through something right now in life that could be throwing your healing journey off just a bit? Are you stressed about money? Life is busy with all sorts of stuff to worry about, so ponder on ways to lessen that worry or stress and I bet the perfect temporary or permanent solutions will reveal themselves soon.

⟿

Now that I have provided a glimpse into emotional and behavioral responses while trying to heal from any physical condition, I want to stress the fact that if we repeat the same bad behaviors over and over, we are not helping ourselves. The final resolution needs to come when we accept change and accept that we are "special" and need to live a "special" life, and we are willing to do what it takes. This is not all bad. Once you realize, commit, and overcome—which I call the restoration phase—your life is going to open you up to more opportunities and more love than you could have ever imagined. It's sometimes through the bad that we discover the best.

In Dr. Pagano's book, he mentions a patient with Ps who ate red meat and tomatoes every day of his life; he even told Dr. Pagano he ate tomatoes by the bushel. The only time his Ps ever disappeared was when he was hospitalized for several weeks after a heart attack. The doctors and even him were baffled as to why his Ps went away. When he was released, he returned home and continued to eat his same diet. His Ps came back with a vengeance. It turns out, red meat and tomatoes were not intravenously fed to him during that time. He was excited to start working with Dr. Pagano on the diet, but unfortunately, he passed away before they could begin.

The reason I share this story is not to shock you, it is because I want to inspire you to make the change now. When I read this story, everything inside of me wanted to stay on track because I want to live and be happy. Reading stories about others or watching all the documentaries you can to learn about those who have suffered and succeeded often motivates us to try harder.[30]

I understand that it all depends on where you are at with your life and your condition. I don't know about you, but I was desperate and ready to commit. I was chatting with a friend of a friend once who had huge patches of Ps all over her body. You would think she'd be ready, but she adamantly said to me, "I will not live life without my coffee and tomatoes." When I asked her how much of these she eats and how often, she proceeded to tell me she drinks five cups of coffee every morning and eats two huge fresh tomatoes for lunch every day. It turns out she was raised eating freshly sliced tomatoes daily with her lunch; it's what she knows and loves. I understand her resistance to giving it up, but I would rather not live with Ps.

We are all ready at different stages and have different comfort levels. You can choose to eat whatever you want; it's your body. But, if you are ready to heal, you will change. For me, I had to hit rock bottom and feel done living with Ps. I had to

---

30   There are lots of resources in the bibliography and also on my website.

look at my behavior and try not to repeat the same behaviors over and over again. Try to look at where you might be, and if you're aware that your behavior or diet or lifestyle is not helping, do something about it. Take action! If you absolutely need your coffee, and life isn't worth living without it, then simply cut down or try mixing some decaffeinated in it. If you can't live without pizza, try white cheese pizza. That's what I do when I'm in a situation where everyone is ordering pizza for dinner and I'm not the one catering. I just ask if they can order me a slice or two of the white cheese pizza. Pizza is a very acidic concoction, so I eat it rarely, but I'm giving you an example. At the beginning of my journey, I wouldn't even eat pizza; I would just eat before leaving the house, or I'd bring something to eat and explain it to my friends ahead of time. But now my journey is very different. My skin is healed for the most part, and I eat stuff like that sparingly.

So, with having looked at our emotional and behavioral responses, what does this restoration phase look like, and what is included in these new behaviors?

Let me start by reiterating that when you are repairing your skin from the inside out you are giving yourself the greatest gift: to receive love from you! What is a life without love, patience, acceptance, and freedom in your skin? It's not a very joyful one, is it? When I think of patience, I think of standing in a long line somewhere when it's the last place you want to be. It's one of the most difficult things to learn to do, to suffer in some way while you manage not to let it get you upset or angry. I happen to be a very patient person, which I feel very grateful for. My husband, not so much! I was recently a passenger in a car on a long ride. While the driver was getting extremely agitated at the traffic and slow drivers,

I was feeling appreciative of my gift of patience. I just don't let long waits bother me (unless there is a true emergency!). If I'm going for a long ride, I will expect it to be a good one, traffic or no traffic. So, when it came to healing my skin and reading about patience in Dr. Pagano's book (he urges you to find it), I was ready. It took me an entire year to heal myself at first, but I knew it would take some time, and I mentally prepared myself for it. That's what I suggest you do, too—prepare yourself mentally for a journey that could take months, or a year, or more. However long it takes, be fine with it and promise to be good to yourself during that time.

Once you accept that it might take some time, you won't be so upset if it does take that long. I have a friend with Ps in Australia, and her patience is always getting tested. She has hair loss, vitiligo, arthritis, and Ps lesions. She is constantly eating clean all while trying to live her life. When her hair was not doing very well, she decided to be really strict with her diet and, during that year, she would always end her emails with a positive statement about how she was hanging in there and knows she's on the right track, or that she knows she's doing the best she could for her body and will continue to find patience during that time. She stayed positive even though, deep down, it was difficult. I cannot express enough how far your positivity will take you. Expect healing! Believe healing will happen for you!

Acceptance was a hard one for me during my journey, but I must tell you, now I stop and think, "Am I accepting where I am at with that negative thought?" I know the best thing we could all do is to accept where we are at and stop torturing ourselves by refusing to accept it. I have a friend who hates her weight. She's always complaining and looking for quick fixes.

I tell her the same thing I'm telling you, but about your skin. You are not going to heal overnight, just like she's not going to lose weight overnight. The best thing to do is accept where you are right now. Just sit with it. Sit with your skin and look at it and know it takes some time, but believe that it will heal.

Whatever you do, do not complain about it; complaining will only enforce the negative and that doesn't serve you or your skin. Freedom is what comes from patience and acceptance. It's the ultimate gift and life will never feel so good without it! I'll never forget the day I went to work with zero Ps on my elbows for the first time. I wore a t-shirt for the first time that summer, and I would pop into the bathroom every now and again to check and make sure it hadn't come back. I didn't know life without it and, boy, was it incredible. Living a life without feeling less than, feeling more whole, not caring what people thought, not worrying that people would see, wanting a man to touch my skin, not having anything in my way — that was the big one. Nothing was in my way of being happy! (I look so forward to you contacting me to tell me how your newfound freedom feels to you. Words cannot express how excited I am for that.)

You have to be ready to make changes in your life, and you have to find the motivation to experiment so you can figure out what works for you; that's the restoration phase. It's easy to say it, but putting it into action? Not so easy. I keep my focus on how I'm feeling, and if I'm feeling good, I know I'm doing something right that my skin will appreciate. For the first time, you will learn to feel in tune with your body.

And, one of the most amazing side effects? You will start to crave better and healthier foods and forget about all the crap you have eaten in the past. It's amazing when I look back to the food I used to crave, like Doritos and chicken nuggets from McDonald's. What I've noticed the most is how much my body doesn't crave those processed foods anymore. I now crave fruit, nuts, and fresh veggies because my body thrives when I give it nutrients. Those nutrients fill me up and help my body run more efficiently than ever before. Yours will, too. I promise! I know you don't believe me yet, but you will see. You will feel so good, so light—you will have so much clarity, and so much energy, that you will naturally want to continue eating healthier. You will feel full! You may not think so, but eating whole foods means you can eat when you're hungry and stop when you're full, and you don't feel a need to eat beyond that, whereas with something like a bag of chips, you just can't stop!

Another wonderful side effect is that you are eating richer, better foods, and you don't gain weight; it's liberating! You also develop good habits. When I need to, I make grains and squashes on Sundays to eat throughout the week, and it saves me money and time. I try to find healthy snacks I can cook, such as roasted chickpeas, kale chips, or sweet potato fries instead of mindlessly buying bags of chips. I remember having my first Dorito at a party about two years into my healing journey, and it tasted like cardboard to me! I would *never* have said that about Doritos years ago; they were my ultimate go-to snack! I could eat half a bag in one sitting! I *loved* them!

It amazes me now how bad processed food tastes compared to real whole foods from the earth, the ones our bodies were intended to eat. I no longer experience bloating, gas, or any discomfort, when, before, that's all I used to feel. You might think you can never live without something, but your body will forget because it is not part of your healing process any longer and, therefore, not important. I had such a hard time saying goodbye to coffee at first, and in my mind, it wasn't for forever. It was temporary while I healed. But now, five years later, I'm stronger, and my body is happier when I drink one of my delicious replacements. When I do have a cappuccino or latte once a year or so, I always get a headache. I bet when you go back to that favorite snack after not having it for a while, it will not taste the same. I talk to so many people who tell me how surprised they are by this. One woman was shocked at how sweet a refined, processed pastry tasted after fruit being her go-to sugar for six months. She had eaten those pastries for breakfast every day, and now she can't eat them anymore; she prefers her mixed fresh fruit.

So, trust me, you will make it through your craving, you will find satisfying replacements, and you will move forward into loving and craving healthy, delicious whole foods. Through actively working and managing your needs and likes ahead of time, you will never feel deprived. And it is deprivation that stops any diet short in its tracks. But a food lifestyle change will release all of that, and you will find foods you just love, and they will love you back.

⬱

To help you understand what restoration looks like, I am sharing a few key words, phrases and concepts that you can use as a go-to when you are feeling stuck. Just come back and read these sections when you need some redirection.

Help Yourself Receive

To illustrate the concept of helping yourself receive, here was one of my journaling exercises:

Universe, help me receive! I have been struggling with my acting career and feeling like giving up. I am being pulled toward this health path and wanting to help hundreds of people and make a contribution to the world somehow. I think I thought acting was going to be the way to contribute, to move people in some way, to make them feel something, but now I'm seeing it's this other health path that seems to be moving me the most. I'm struggling with trying to figure out exactly what I'm here to do in that arena, and I would like you to help point me in the right direction to a career that will be the most fulfilling, rewarding, loving, helpful, and exciting experience for me. I want to wake up excited to start my day! Show me universe...I'm listening, and looking....

The feeling in me was a torn feeling, because I didn't like thinking of myself as giving up, and I don't want people to think I gave up on my acting. I feel like I went through this with my production career. Giving it up felt hard, and I was scared of judgment—maybe more of my judgment than anyone else's, but now I look at it as growth. Growing nets a career and life that is rewarding and nourishing and one that you can enjoy every day. Isn't this where you want to be?

Don't worry, common feelings we all experience include: *What will people think? How can I change direction again? What am I doing here?* Put the questions out to the universe, and then take your time to listen. You will be very surprised at the opportunities that open in your new path.

Patience

"Patience is a virtue," is the old saying. I'm learning, at my ripe old age of forty that it *really* is. I was emailing recently with a new friend who has Ps about patience because he's having a hard time. He's taking good care of himself and has been for months, and has seen progress, but it's slow going and, while one area is clearing, another is popping up. It frustrates me to hear that, for two reasons. First, because he's truly doing everything he can not to put acidic foods in his body and he's doing a load of healthy things on a daily basis like yoga, baths, etc. Second, this alkaline lifestyle is working so well for me, so why not him? I know we all are different with different bodies and thought processes, so I try to keep that in mind, but it's hard hearing news like this and makes me want to come to the rescue and figure it out. I feel stress has a bigger part to play than even food, and I firmly believe the more you worry about something, the more you will see it in your life. So, I'm hoping he finds a way not to focus and stress over it as much as he is. It's hard. Trust me, I know!

This is where patience comes in. It's such an essential thing, isn't it? In Dr. Pagano's book, it's amazing to read about the dozens of cases he had where some people cleared in five months and some took over a year. When I struggled with a small patch on my leg after eight months, and even though it cleared a little each day, it was still there, and I paid attention to it. It was hard to see beyond it.

These are the times for positive affirmations. I've made a conscious choice to focus on the positive: most of my Ps is gone, and this patch is fading. It's taking time, but it is fading and not reappearing. I'm well aware that by focusing on the positive results I'm not a prisoner to my ego, which likes to focus on the negative. I'm patient because, although it has taken time, it *is* leaving. I'm patient because I've had Ps for over twenty-one years and I know it's not going to exit overnight. I'm patient because I know I'm doing right by my body through eating and exercise and thinking good thoughts. I'm patient because I know there's no other choice than to be patient or be miserable. I also know that this patience will lead to a longer and healthier life.

What do you choose? Sit down and ask yourself where your focus is. It's not easy to focus on the positive aspects of your Ps when you are looking right at it. I know that, and in no way do I want you to think it is easy. I just know nothing felt better than taking my life back by choosing not to let my Ps control me. I'm patient because I love myself enough to be happy!

Acceptance

You know that saying, "You want what you don't have"? Well, when I was younger, I'd find myself always wanting what other people had. Maybe it was straight hair, or a nicer car, or a wealthier family, or a cute boyfriend—the list goes on and on. Of course at the top of my list: other people's clear skin. I'd watch people showing lots of skin in short jean shorts and tank tops and be so envious. I'd daydream of what it felt like to not have a complex about my skin! What must that feel like? No, really, what must that feel like to live life with no insecurity about your skin? I just couldn't imagine, but I really, really, wanted to know. I felt people took their clear skin for granted and, if I were them, I would flaunt my skin every day and feel proud of it and show it to the world and love it. I was dying to love it. I just wanted to buy a fun pair of shorts and feel good in them.

As I got older, I found myself becoming more accepting of my life and more grateful for the abundance I have. I guess that comes with maturity. I found myself wanting to start feeling proud of my skin even if it disappointed me. I wanted to appreciate it because it was mine and it was going to be with me forever. Acceptance is such an interesting and difficult thing, and it snuck up on me in my thirties. I resisted feeling thankful for my skin my whole life and, one day, something shifted, and I started to want to accept myself more. I didn't want to hide anymore.

My friends and family all have their ailments and issues. Some have bad eyesight, some are overweight, some underweight…teeth issues, diabetes, fatigue, allergies, depression, addiction, narcissism, control issues, the list goes on. My point is that we all have something we struggle with, whether it's psychological and emotional, or physical, and we can't help but compare ourselves to others sometimes. We all would rather have their issue than our own sometimes. I said "sometimes." I always thought I'd be fine swapping anybody's issue for mine, but I don't think that way anymore. I was meant to have Ps because I was meant to go down this healthy road and discover all this wonderful information and bring it to others. And you know what? I've never felt more fulfilled and healthier. That's how I know it was meant to be!

Acceptance is such a beautiful thing because it produces confidence. Feeling confident feels so good, right? It's even more attractive in other people. Think about it, who would you rather hang out with? A confident person who feels good about themselves and is genuinely happy and loving, or an insecure person who is down all the time, unhappy, and constantly complaining? I'm sure if I was complaining in this book about how bad life was with Ps and woe is me, you probably wouldn't read it. I wouldn't! I do everything I can to surround myself with positive, happy people who contribute something wonderful to my life. They give me inspiration, love, and joy.

I make it a point to try to be kind and loving to everyone in life, because I feel that's what life is about. I also believe that my Ps has stayed away because there is less stress in my life after bidding farewell to some negative people who played big parts in it these last few years. My skin craves positive energy. It's pretty amazing what happens when you start consciously acting more kind and loving—it comes back to you. It really does! I'm not just referring to others; I'm also talking about your relationship with your body. If you are good to your body, it'll be good to you.

I want to inspire people to be more grateful for their journey instead of cursing it. Ask yourself why you are on this journey. Make love your intention. Setting intentions is very powerful! Just because we have Ps doesn't make us bad, ugly, or not enough. We can feel empowered in our skin if we want to, but it's just easier to surrender to self-loathing. Why? Why is it easier to complain about something going wrong in our lives than to focus on the lesson from it and turn it into a positive? Maybe we love the drama? I know I sometimes do, but there is a time and place for everything.

Just take a moment before reacting to that negative thought with another negative thought and say to yourself, "This doesn't need to be a negative thing. There is always something positive about everything." Then, point out one positive thing about it. It's a start!

Here's an example:

Negative: "I hate my skin! Why do I have the ugliest skin disease ever? It makes me feel so ugly!"

Positive: "If I didn't have this disease, I most likely wouldn't have gone down this healthy road and wouldn't be as healthy and clean as I am today. Thanks to my condition I found this new lifestyle, and I feel amazing! I appreciate my Ps leading the way down this path of wellness!"

I'm sure some of you are totally rolling your eyes right now. I know how hard it is to love yourself when you have Ps. It's damn hard, but it's your choice to try. Try to love yourself. If you make the positive choice, I guarantee you will see amazing results in how you feel day to day.

A raw food chef named Dara Dubinet (famous for her YouTube channel on raw food videos, and who has a great one on inflammation and leaky gut) said she looks at any health issue as a health *opportunity* that is there to give her a wake-up call her body clearly needs.[31] Is that not brilliant, or what? Go back and read that again. That is the exact point of view I want to have forever. She interviewed a man named Joe Cross from the film, *Fat, Sick and Nearly Dead*, who said his new motto is "change equals opportunity." Ps changed my life for the better; it can change yours too.

---

31 Dara Dubinet, "What is leaky gut and how to fix inflammation with raw food & ginger juice" *(sic)*: https://youtu/jPgFKmuF0nE.

A while after writing this and thinking about my journey, a word came to me, and it was "freedom." I realize freedom is all we really want. This started changing my perspective and how I viewed things. I own that I choose to make poor choices here and there because I like certain foods that don't like me and, at the end of the day, I just want to be able to eat whatever the heck I want. I want freedom with food, even if that means eating whatever I wanted even if it was bad for me—until I started to think more deeply about this process and realized that that was not freedom, that was a food craving or need that controlled me.

I had to ask myself why I didn't feel freedom when it came to food. On my journey, I continue to come back to this question: why? I realized I used food my whole life to feel safe and in control. In all my chaotic environments, it was the one thing I could control—whether it was as a child growing up in a dysfunctional home, working in TV where the environment was crazy and stressful, or chasing my dream to act, which was completely unpredictable. I also dated emotionally unavailable men until I was thirty-seven and finally met my husband. I tended to want control wherever I could get it, and food was that weapon for me.

Sometimes, when we can't change a situation or circumstance, we look for something we *can* change. Food numbed me when I needed it to, it made me feel alive when I needed it to, and it made me feel I had some control when I needed it to. The problem was, that control grew into something that made me feel more guilt and shame, just like I felt with my Ps. I love food, and I want to enjoy it, not have it be something that makes me feel bad when I think about it or eat it.

So when I say I want freedom from food, what I'm saying is, I don't want to feel like I have to have control with it, like I did in all those other aspects of my life. I'm ready to let go and allow life to be simpler. I gave food a deeper meaning than just looking at it as a means to live a healthy, vibrant life. I'm aware now, and my psychological struggle is coming to an end.

A lot of us have restrictions and judgments when it comes to feeding ourselves. I wouldn't want anyone reading this book to force themselves to eat well. I would want you to become aware of how you look at food, how you might use it in a way that satisfies some deep, dark, emotional place in you. Become aware, and then be loving and kind to yourself now that you know. There isn't a time when you completely arrive and, suddenly, you're a master of feeling freedom from food, but once you find ways to be kind to yourself, listen to your body more, and look at it as your friend, you *will* feel freer!

One of the most amazing things (that will take time for you to appreciate) is that you will come to enjoy your time eating healthy, and even the stuff you eat or prepare will become a flavor and a moment to appreciate. I truly enjoy my green juice and the veggies and beans. But if I'm out, and running errands, and the healthiest convenient place to stop for lunch isn't quite ideal, I just want to be able to stop and eat a delicious wrap or salad and soup. I don't want to think about what's in it that I can't have. In the old days, I was angry and sick of thinking about food, now I have the freedom of 90/10 and don't worry about it.

I know it feels like you are carrying the largest burden of your life with Ps, and everyone handles things differently. For me, thinking and preparing food for my typical work week isn't that terrible for the most part. For you, the thought of shopping, thinking, planning, and prepping might turn you off and make you want to run in the opposite direction.

The big question I'm trying to answer here is: How does someone with a skin disease — or, honestly, anyone dealing with any disease — feel freedom enough to enjoy their new healing lifestyle through food?

I want to share some answers I find helpful. There is not necessarily a right or wrong here; it is more about adopting the idea to fit what gives you freedom. The truth is, freedom means different things to different people, but when it comes to illness, most people want to be free of it. It may surprise you but, psychologically, some people like to hold on to their illness because it brings them attention and sympathy. If this rings true for you, then it is worth exploring the benefits of giving up the illness for health and how you will attain positive attention versus negative. I intend to discuss this more in my next book and my workshops, but it's too much to get into here. Start simple with these two recommendations:

1. Find food replacements or substitutes to conquer the craving before they hit and keep your options in your house or with you. You must have some go-to replacements that are *enjoyable*. Giving up coffee was tough, and I knew I wasn't going to last if I didn't find some hot beverage that would satisfy my coffee fix. It was not just the taste of it either; I loved carrying it as I walked around the city on my way to work. It became my morning routine, and I looked so forward to it. Change is hard, but you have to be open to change if you want to see a change in your life. I felt lucky and excited when

I found decaf chai tea, Teeccino, and Dandy Blend, all of which helped replace the "feel" of the coffee experience.

2. Find a way not to beat yourself up if you backtrack. Every day is a process, every day is a new start, and as they say in AA, take one day at a time.

We are all challenged at times. If you start to go in the direction of poor choices, it is probably time to have a talk with yourself. You can remind yourself that this is one meal out of many healthier ones and that it's not the end of the world if a meal or snack here and there isn't on your diet.

Sometimes, I'll have to talk myself into making the better choice. Sometimes you just have to go off track. I'm sorry, but you do. You can't live life feeling deprived. Life is meant to be joyful and, I don't know about you, but I need to feel the joy of splurging now and again. The truth is, I don't feel that guilty about it at the moment; it's when my skin is being stubborn that I do, because I know it'll just prolong the desired goal of clearing.

I try to make the best choices and decisions, and most of the time these days, I do. When you do, too, pat yourself on the back and say, "I'm proud of you." It's worth focusing on. People are so quick to focus on the negative aspect of everything. Why is that? We have a choice of focusing on the positive or negative, and if our focus on the positive makes us feel good, then why anything else? I used to focus on the negative of situations because, on some level, it made me feel safe. It's silly if you think about it. Shouldn't we do or think about what makes us feel good? Always?

I believe that if you don't give so much attention to the things that upset you, they will get better. This gives you emotional freedom. The more we pay attention to things and complain about them, the more we reinforce them. I think deep down in our unconscious somewhere, we feel good having something to complain about, something to vent about to friends and strangers. My question is why? Why do we feel compelled to focus on what's not working for us and make it worse by complaining and worrying and stressing about it all day, every day? I can't help but think, on some level, it makes us feel comforted or safe in some way. Are we scared to feel nothing but happiness and joy?

My entire life, I never felt appreciation for my body. I either felt nothing, or shame. My journey has brought me to this place of appreciation, with or without Ps patches. It took a long time to get here, and I might feel frustration sometimes, but deep down I know in my bones that my body is doing the best it can and I have to show it love for that. If we hate our weight, our skin, or our shape, we will be shown more things to hate. If we feel appreciation for the healthy foods we are eating, for the healthy oil we are applying, and focus on the parts we like, we will start to see more to like. That is everything: picking the parts you like, glorifying them, and the others will one day not feel so important. Your emotional response to them will be released, and you will live a much happier life. As Elizabeth A. Behnke said, "There is deep wisdom in our flesh if we can only come to our senses and feel it."

❦

Ps: Really *feel* your feelings, validate them, know they came into your life for a reason, and be willing to release the ones that no longer serve a positive purpose in your life, because your skin craves positive attention.

Meditation

Right now I'm feeling _____ (fill in the blank). I accept where I am at right now. I accept these feelings of _____ right now in this moment. Take a deep breath; breathe that feeling in and breathe it out. When you exhale, breathe it out through your mouth and imagine that feeling leaving your body along with it. Thank it for coming for whatever purpose it has in protecting you. Continue to breathe and release it. Tell yourself you are in the restoration phase and have already realized, committed, and overcome. By the time you come out of the meditation, tell yourself you are *restored*! Consciously create images in your mind that express what freedom is to you and tell yourself you love yourself so much that when you come out of the meditation, you will manifest this change, and it will be easier than you ever imagined possible. You are now free.

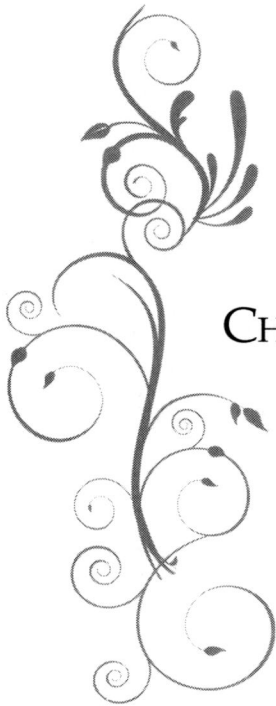

Chapter Ten

Self-Love: The Final Key

*I am worth healing. I am
worth the time it takes to learn
how to nourish myself.
I love you, body.*

Louise Hay

SELF-LOVE IS:	SELF-LOVE IS NOT:
• Spending quality time with yourself and doing what brings you joy.	• Beating yourself up when you mess up.
• Being loving and kind to yourself in any way, shape, or form.	• Criticizing yourself or others.
• Putting yourself first before anyone else.	• Judging yourself or others.
• Making your health a priority.	• Sabotaging yourself and your progress because you are hurt or angry.
• Trusting things are going to work out and taking risks.	• Thinking negatively.
• Doing what lights you up inside and chasing your dreams.	• Keeping emotions bottled up.
• Being who you are and not who others want you to be.	• Being self-destructive.

• Believing in yourself.	• Attacking others when you are angry at yourself.
• Trusting yourself.	• Just accepting a doctor's opinion because they are a doctor.
• Wanting the best for yourself and others.	• Eating and drinking or taking modified, concocted, mass-produced products without thinking hard or doing your research to learn what is really in them.
• Genuinely loving yourself, not hating yourself.	• Taking medications without doing your research to learn what is really in them.
• Forgiving yourself and others.	• Lying to yourself about who you really are.
• Appreciating and being grateful for all that's around us and in our lives.	• Picking on every little part of your being you don't like.
• Loving your body even when it makes you feel less than.	• Thinking you can do and handle it all perfectly.
• Figuring out ways to de-stress.	• Pushing unconditional love away because you have never had it before.
• Finding your voice and standing up for yourself.	
• Living your life with purpose and meaning.	
• Nourishing your body with real food.	
• Living and relaxing by enjoying the right now moment.	
• Accepting help when so many people have willing hearts.	

As I discussed in the previous chapter, I know that insecurity, shame, and fear are involved in having psoriasis with lesions or spots that are visible on your skin. It's intense and hard because people can see them and they judge; and when they judge you, you feel insecure and not good enough. I know that emotions of all kinds play a huge factor in what is going on in our lives, in our bodies, and in our spirits. And I have come to realize that I don't think too many people love themselves enough to do all the loving things they can do to heal, because they are missing this one final piece.

As we near the conclusion of the book, and if you have stuck with me this far, I need you to stay with me until the end to get this life-changing information. All of this research and learning by trial and error has led up to what I believe is one of the most crucial steps in the healing process, from all diseases and conditions, and it is something that I feel most people have not given enough attention. This component of your healing has so much more influence than most people would ever realize. It is an aspect of our journey that demands we make time for ourselves, a component that says we need to acknowledge our real emotions and find the source of our fears and rejections. It demands that we come to the table open-hearted and make friends with ourselves and all our weaknesses, not just our strengths. In the end, it's what teaches us unconditional love and makes us who we are.

Without further delay, that one component, that one key to access health, that one final missing puzzle piece is... self-love.

Self-love is such an interesting concept, because it is not something that can be defined easily or in a few words. Self-love is something we work to achieve. It is something we think of or see in saints and charitable beings. It is because they have accepted and loved themselves to the highest level that they can give this to others easily and matter-of-factly without a thought, and without ever feeling used. Because you may have never realized the importance of this before — and it took me almost forty years — I am going to try to teach you what that means by using episodes in my life and by providing examples of what it does not mean.

Some of these points and stories may seem so very obvious up front, but when you scratch a little deeper below the surface, you start to realize the behaviors and attitudes that led up to them may mean you are sabotaging yourself. So, let me begin with some examples and stories of what self-love is *not*, to make my point, then provide a little lesson on how to improve so that you can become your best and healed self.

🐚

Self-love is not leaving your food options to other people, but is caring enough about yourself always to be prepared.

Lesson: In an ideal world other people are just as caring for you as you are for them, but you can't take it personally if they don't prepare for your dietary restrictions.

This is one of the hard lessons I learned along the way, and it happened while I was acting. I had somehow been taught to believe and even expect that in this new world of people with allergies, assorted intolerances, and other dietary requirements, I could get what I needed for food wherever I was, especially in my profession where it was provided to save time because you were always on the job.

I was shooting a short film, and it was a rough schedule. In two days we had worked a total of thirty-eight hours: twenty hours the first day and eighteen the second. When working on independent low-budget projects, you can't expect they will always provide healthy meals or snack options. I now know to bring a bunch of healthy snacks with me in case I get hungry, to avoid craft service, which on this kind of shoot is usually not much more than bagels and cookies.

In this particular instance, I found myself in a bit of a pickle. They ordered lunch without asking anyone about food restrictions. So, here we are at someone's house, and the caterer comes in, drops off sandwiches and potato salad, and off they go. I was very excited because I was starving and a veggie sandwich sounded perfect to me. I was even going to eat it on white bread, just not to be too much of a diva.

We broke for lunch, and I slowly realized that the entire sandwich platter was meat. You can imagine the horror on my face and in my belly. How could a whole team of people not have thought to ask anyone if they didn't eat meat? I was baffled by this and didn't know what to do. I considered asking the director if someone could drive me so I could get my own lunch, but this was an "eat fast and get back to work" lunch because we were so far behind schedule.

I decided to eat the Lara bar and apple I had in my bag and planned on requesting veggie sandwiches the following day. A few people saw me eating my apple and felt terrible for me after I explained why. I felt disappointed in the crew for not meeting my expectations.

I learned if other people aren't thinking of my food restrictions, then I need to be. I thought about this the whole way home that night, starving, and realized I couldn't trust other people to take care of my needs the way I trust myself to. I could have emailed the director a week before to make sure he was aware, but I just trusted there would be options for vegetarians. Lesson learned. Now, the question is, can you fend for yourself and be prepared and not feel hurt when others don't "cater" to you? Life is a give and take, but if we are prepared and have realistic expectations, we won't be so surprised if something doesn't go our way. Love yourself enough always to be prepared. It will save you a lot of disappointment, and you will eat healthier.

🙊

Self-love is not beating yourself up.

Lesson: Be supportive and kind to yourself even when you don't like what you see.

During my early journey, I found I would beat myself up if my Ps didn't fade fast enough. I'm sure, like most Ps sufferers, when you are spot-free you feel in control and great; but at other times, when spots emerge, your first reaction is to feel defeated again. One time, right after a few spots had re-emerged, I found myself at home with Mike, saying, "Why isn't it going away faster? I'm working so hard!" Mike's response was priceless. He said, "Kim, it's only been two weeks." I said, "Oh yeah, you're right!"

It felt like I had a mini-epiphany at that moment. He was so right. It had been only the first two weeks of my journey, so why was I already punishing myself? Why was I already feeling I had failed? Why did my brain go right to the negative? This made me think a lot about why we talk so badly to ourselves. I thought about what I'd say to a close friend. I know I'd be supportive and loving and remind her that it's a marathon, not a sprint, tell her she was beautiful inside and out. So, why wouldn't I say that to myself?

I want you to think about this, because real self-love is un-conditionally loving yourself every minute of every day, with the good, the bad, and the ugly! How does it serve us to beat ourselves up and talk negatively to ourselves? Think about the impact and how we feel after someone has cut us down or been negative or mean to us. Therefore, how do you feel af-ter telling yourself you are not doing well enough? Like crap, that's how.

The question is: Why do we engage in negative self-talk? Why aren't we nicer and more loving toward ourselves? Instead of saying, "Why doesn't my skin look better, I'm kill-ing myself here?" the key is to turn the negative thoughts in a positive direction, even if it is just a small one, and say some-thing as simple as, "My skin takes time to clear, and I will be patient. I am doing the best I can. Good job! I am trying. I can and will succeed."

This journey has led me to spend a lot of time wondering why our minds naturally go to that negative place, because I don't like that one bit. I have made a conscious decision to focus more on changing my negative thoughts to positive ones, and it's hard as can be. I'm naturally a positive person. If you met anyone in my life, they would describe me as hap-py and positive. So, if I'm so naturally positive, why does my brain insist on going to that dark place? These are questions I started giving a lot of thought to and decided I had to learn a way to re-program my thoughts, because I needed to live a happy life, with or without Ps. I am encouraging you just to try this out and observe how you feel when you do it. You may feel uncomfortable at first, like you're lying to yourself, but eventually, you realize you are being nicer to yourself, and it feels natural and right, and it will turn the direction in a positive way toward healing.

Remember, it would be impossible for anyone to ignore a medical condition that affects their life, and I'm not asking you to be in denial. What I am asking is that, when you see it, when it presents itself, to not focus negatively on it. This is not easy. I wish I could not pay attention to the progress of my Ps, but it's hard to ignore and not check on it every minute of the day. I highly recommend that first, you limit how often you look to no more than two times a day, and instead of fretting and freaking, clear your mind and pretend you are healed, or that you have already reached your goal.

A perfect example of the mind—because, as humans, we have such an issue with delayed gratification—is when we go on a diet and think if we step on the scale ten times a day we will see something different. Everyone knows that if you step on the scale throughout the day, because of water retention or simply using a different scale, the results could be different each time. But if we just started a diet or started working out, then why are we already saying to ourselves, "How come I haven't lost any weight?" When we can't immediately visually see something, we start to complain, "Why is everything so hard for me? Why isn't this working? What's wrong with me?" You know the drill.

I do check my spots (or where they were) in the morning and at night, but I know, deep down, I'm better off not looking at all. When you eat so clean, you do think it should go away in a few days or weeks. Patience is so hard to have, whether you are experiencing something on the outside for everyone to see, or you know you have cancer or a medical illness that is attacking you from the inside. The most important piece is being kind and loving to yourself, and expecting the best, but not pressuring or sabotaging yourself if you don't see it that second. So, no matter what, be supportive and kind to yourself, even if you don't like what you see.

ᘒ

Self-love is not expecting the great results others have all the time and realizing there are many people who have it so much harder, so who are you to feel picked on?

Lesson: Learn to love your individual journey and honor it — it's what makes you special.

I have also learned that the healing journey is completely individual, so what has worked for me might not work for you. I wish it were one-size-fits-all, but unfortunately, it isn't. For example, at the beginning of my journey, I stayed away from all things acidic, but now I have them 10 percent of the time without it affecting my Ps. That may not be the case for you. You may need to eliminate acidic foods first, then slowly incorporate them back in while monitoring your progress. That's what I did. But with foods like eggs, I never saw a difference and my Ps continued to heal. As a result, I know I can have eggs and chicken here and there and still be fine.

We each have a unique journey that's trying to teach us something. My lesson is to love myself more, with or without Ps. To do that, I know I can't compare myself to others. I say this knowing it is tough not to compare when you see someone with perfect, clear, glowing skin walking around in short shorts without a care in the world. You want that more than anything, I know. I did, too, for many years. What I'm trying to get you to understand is, the more you give yourself compliments on the things you do like, the more you will start to see things you like — things you might have missed before because you were focusing on being critical versus being loving.

I might have a spot of Ps on my calf, but I truly love my calves. They are perfect to me when my skin is clear, and now I can love them even when I am not totally clear! So I try my best to focus on this aspect of me I like and do notice my calves looking better and better. I can now enjoy them even with a few minor imperfections.

I know that this is not easy, especially when we all play the comparison game to some degree. We all know those women with the perfect metabolism, the perfect skin, who don't seem to age, who have all the perfect genes. We all know advertising makes us feel we have to look like we should be in *Vogue*. But you forget all the make-up and photo-brushing and Photoshopping that goes on. Do you believe people wake up in the morning looking like that? Do you believe that the mascara ads do what they say they do and that there are not falsies on those eyelashes as well?

I always advise never to compare yourself to anyone else. They are not as good as they may seem because every human has a component that they struggle with, and no human is perfectly crafted to be a hundred percent beautiful to everyone. Why do you think some love blondes, some brunettes, some Asians, some fair-skinned, and so on? Diversity is good! So stop comparing and just dive in and start figuring out what you can complement yourself on, and do what you need to do for you and your beloved body to heal. Love your individual journey and honor it. It is truly what makes you unique and special.

Self-love is not believing you are the only person in the world who this has ever happened to or has ever suffered and that it could never be worse.

Lesson: It can always be worse. Learn to honor those around you and realize how many people who suffer in far worse situations than yours. Don't be hard on yourself. Instead, appreciate the good things you have.

Often, we get so wrapped up in ourselves that we forget there are people suffering more than we are. What I have noticed in my journey is that when I feel bad, I tend to reach out to others who are also feeling bad — others who are often doing worse than me, maybe have worse skin than me — and it honestly humbles me and makes me want to help them more. Helping them makes me feel better. I've had Ps for over twenty years. It's a long time to feel such negativity about your body — the shame, embarrassment, and insecurity. You should love your body, right? It's a big part of you! I do have to say, though, despite how much I suffered from Ps, I do feel very grateful to have it mildly compared to other people. I've been on the public forums, read books, seen pictures, and my heart breaks for all the people suffering out there. From open wounds to lesions on the face to scarring to loss of hair due to issues with the scalp, you name it. And on top of that, Ps is not even a terminal illness. It may feel like it, but it is not. So, for that, we should all take a moment to say thanks. Take a moment and thank the universe, because this is something you can overcome. Appreciate the good things you have going for you, because you could always have it worse.

Self-love is NOT trusting doctors and professional advice more than you trust yourself.

Lesson: Respect your doctors, learn from your doctors, but make sure you get a doctor who takes time and communicates with you — or get a new doctor. Do your research and don't settle, because you and your life are way too valuable.

I find our entire medical mentality sad. Medications are made up of toxic chemicals. I know they may be needed depending on the illness, and they can indeed help with pain. (Heaven knows I've had my fair share of accidents!) However, I can't help but know in my gut that dependence on medication will only make us worse over time. And although this is a topic for an entirely different book, I want to talk about the professionals, the doctors that administer these medications.

We all value an expert opinion. Let's face it, we feel better when a person has letters after their name. We feel more comfortable that they have strong credentials, and we feel safe taking direction from those people. But at the end of the day, my dermatologist didn't heal my skin, I did.

I am learning that we are our own best doctors. Who knows our body better than we do? Obviously, we need doctors for lots of important reasons. But if we listen to our bodies more, we might be able to figure it out ourselves without medications. If I had kept taking my dermatologist's advice, I'd still be allowing Ps to control me with medications that thin my skin and fill my bloodstream with toxic chemicals. I hear the same story so often at the Institute for Integrative Nutrition. So many people enroll because they have a loved one who had suffered from a severe illness only to heal it by avoiding the doctor's recommendations and choosing real food along with the power of positive thinking and believing.

One man who spoke at a conference I attended recently said his mother with breast cancer was told by her doctor that if she chose the holistic road and avoided chemotherapy and radiation she'd be dead in one year. She was willing to take that risk after a random massage therapist suggested she change her diet. Fifteen years later she's never felt better. A massage therapist. You read that correctly—not her medical doctor!

Another woman spoke about her thirteen-year battle trying to help her daughter's extreme asthma and how it came to an end when she read online that eliminating eggs and dairy would help. She was crying while telling this story because she and her daughter had spent most of the girl's first thirteen years in the hospital suffering while being prodded and poked instead of playing outside. She had never played outside and, according to the doctors, she never would. She's now well and playing soccer at school. I was crying listening to all the stories, one after the next. I'm crying right now writing this.

In general, my dermatologist isn't a bad person and doctors are not bad people. I'm not bashing them at all. They get into this field to help others get well, and I admire that. The issue is that they don't receive training in diet and lifestyle. It's not their fault. They are trained in how to diagnose and treat a person with medication and sometimes surgery. This has to change if we are going to be a healthy society, not one that relies on doctors and medications. It's a vicious cycle that is not sustainable. We have children who have adult diseases and illnesses. That's just wrong and sad. No child should have Adult Type II diabetes. Change has to come about, and we have to initiate it. We need to start to take control of our own well-being.

One story that is very close to home involves my husband, Mike. Before we met, in his bachelor days, he was a bit too much into having beer and pizza for dinner every night. His blood work showed he had borderline high cholesterol. His doctor said, "I'm going to give you a prescription to lower it." Mike knew deep down that medication wasn't the answer, and he knew all too well there was only so long he could binge on beer and pizza. He passed on the script and told his doctor he was going to watch his diet. The doctor then proceeded to talk him out of it, saying that, because of Mike's age, it was a no-brainer and that he should be on it for prevention of a heart attack. So Mike took the script ... and threw it away on his way out. I asked him why he even took it and didn't just say no. He said he felt bullied into it, and it felt like the easiest thing to do at the time. I was so angry when he told me this story! Honestly, I wanted to punch him in the face — the doctor, not Mike. Mike knew better, but think of all the people who don't and listen to their doctor because "doctor knows best." This guy is a doctor. His whole job is to help people get well, and he's feeding them toxic chemicals for no good reason, ones that will potentially get people sicker. It's just gross! Fast-forward two years: we're now living together, and Mike is drinking green smoothies and juices every morning with me. He went back to get his blood work done, and his levels were perfect! Anyone surprised?

A teacher of mine recently was talking about this similar conversation he had with his doctor about his severe mood swings. He told the doctor he read online that sugar is sometimes the cause of mood swings and wanted his opinion. His doctor snapped at him very firmly and said there was no evidence that food has anything to do with this imbalance. I wish you could hear him imitate his doctor. It was so snarky the

way he said this, as if he was being questioned on his experience and taking it very personally. He pointed out something
fascinating, though: Doctors will say there is an absence of
evidence, but the truth is there is a big difference between
there being an absence of evidence and evidence of absence.

In other words, there might not be evidence, but why? He
pointed out that no one funds these studies because you can't
patent them and you can't get rich off of kale! Well, these days
you probably can by using it to start a smoothie business, but
you get his point, right? Because no one funds these studies,
there is an absence of evidence. It's not that there is no evidence, just that no one has done the studies. So, find a doctor
who believes that diet is an important part of your healing.
You don't need to seek out a holistic doctor who isn't covered
by your plan and costs $1,000 a visit. You can start by having
a conversation with your doctor. How do they make you feel
when you see them? Do they rush you? Do they ask what the
issue is and write you a script first thing? Do they ask how
your diet is? Do they make you feel like they care? If not, find
another one—go online, ask around.

My current doctor believes food is at the root of most disease and always makes it a point to talk to his patients about
their diet. Medication is the last resort. I never even knew this
until I walked into his office one day and saw the Hippocrates
quote on his wall: "Let food be thy medicine and medicine be
thy food." Seeing that made me feel so safe, because he gets
it! He also does something else that a lot of doctors don't do;
he spends time with his patients and talks with them about
what is going on in their lives, their health concerns, lifestyle
choices, etc. Last time I was there for my annual blood work
we chatted for forty-five minutes. I ended up telling him all

about my health journey with psoriasis and that I was going to school for nutrition and becoming a health coach. He was so happy, and I happily took the compliment that I was his prize patient!

Another wonderful part was that instead of hiding behind the veil of his degrees, he talked to me about his life as well. He told me all about his trip to Peru. He told me about how he and his wife adopted a baby and how painful the adoption process was. It was the most fulfilling doctor's appointment I've ever had. I gave him a hug at the end because I was so touched that he wasn't rushing off to the next patient and had made me feel cared for.

This is one of the things that I feel health coaching gives to people that our current healthcare industry doesn't: the ability to be heard without judgment while being guided and supported back to wellness. I expressed to my doctor how much I appreciated him giving me his time and how much he shared and told him this was the first doctor appointment I've ever had where I felt we were building a relationship and that I wasn't on an assembly line. He told me how frustrating it is to adhere to the medical community's guidelines nowadays, which is to see as many patients in one day as possible in ten-minute increments. He chooses to stay late every night to do his notes until 10:00 p.m. so he can have more time with his patients, because that was why he became a doctor—to help people, talk to them, to figure out what is really going on, and how to heal their condition without medication if possible. He said the only way to get to the cause is by talking everything through to find out what's going on in their life. Is work stressful? Family stressful? Diet? Lack of time to exercise? Can you imagine if our health care system was set up to include this?

Personal conversation is missing in our doctor's visits. If a patient is depressed, don't you think your doctor should ask you what's going on in your life? I'm not implying they become a therapist, but maybe through talking about it, you will realize it's a symptom of your toxic relationship or the stress you have in your job or the lack of time you have to do what brings you joy. This is what I love about the Institute for Integrative Nutrition. They teach us about primary food and secondary food. Primary food is healthy relationships, a fulfilling career, exercise, and having a spiritual practice — whatever that is for you. Then there is secondary food, which is the food we put in our mouths. You can eat all the broccoli you want, but if your primary food isn't balanced, then secondary food can't help you heal. The primary food is what nourishes you more than actual food. This is what took me my whole life to learn, and this is what I want to share with you.

By the way, I recently went to my dermatologist for an annual skin check where I ended up telling her all about my journey. She seemed happy for me and asked me some questions about what foods I gave up. I was happy with the session up until the end. After everything I shared with her, she still became a bit pushy about giving me a script to go home with, to have "just in case." I said no thanks a few times and started to feel that gross feeling in my gut that you get when you know someone is trying to rip you off or put you in a vulnerable position to get something from you. It felt horrible, and I couldn't believe she kept pushing it on me. At that moment, I realized why Mike took the script from his doctor and threw it away on his way out. I felt bullied, and from someone I look to for direction on my path to wellness. The only thing is, she's not on my path to wellness and I'll be looking for another dermatologist to get my annual skin checks with each year.

The goal is to take care of you and surround yourself with doctors who believe in what you believe in. Ask around. I'm positive you will hear stories like mine. Then find the perfect doctor. Don't settle. You and your life are way too valuable.

Self-love is not about being perfect with food every time. So you digressed a little...

Lesson: It is about loving yourself enough to get the food choices correct most of the time! Pick yourself up, start again, and allow yourself to be human — because you are.

A surprising discovery or revelation as I made it through the healing journey—and an interesting dichotomy—is that food is not everything.

Recently I was doing an interview, and when the interviewer asked me about my food program, I explained *technically* I don't have one. My program isn't 100 percent "You need to be eating this or that," because what works for me may not work for you. I believe in bio-individuality, and I feel the key is to have them experiment to figure out what makes them feel their best. I guide them and provide suggestions. Then I thought more after he asked the question and realized I'm more of a counselor listening to people while we piece their puzzles together through just talking and having realizations about what needs to change in their lives. It's incredibly rewarding to watch and help them along. It also helps a lot of people to have a guide, a coach, maybe even a little loving watchdog to sneak in that accountability issue and help them realize what they have allowed themselves to sneak away with and is only hurting them.

It's common for people to want the magic pill to lose weight, heal their skin, feel good, and on and on. Life isn't like that, but people don't have patience. And in self-love, you need patience for yourself and others. Everyone wants a shortcut to some degree. They want to make temporary changes to get what they desire, but they don't seem to want to make long-term changes that will give them their best quality of life. I used to be like that, too. After all, I loved my wings and wine or a Guinness, but they are just not worth it to me. They are not worth having these spots on my skin and the feelings that come with it.

This made me think of all these people I've helped all over the world through the Ps forums. One woman's daughter had bad Ps on her face as well as other areas of her body. I remember telling her that I gave up sugar and her reaction about her daughter doing the same was, "Oh no, she loves her cheesecake. There's no way I can take that away from her." It made me think: Why do we allow food to control us? Same thing with a woman I'm helping now; she can't give up caffeine. It's been a long battle, but the coffee always wins. I get it because I used to need my coffee too, but at what price? You will learn that as you begin to care and love yourself and start, little by little, to replace negative foods and emotions with positive ones, it will all become easier, and you will become a kinder, gentler, more self-loving person. The next step? Give up perfection, know you will digress at times, but love yourself and you will find you get back on track more quickly.

Self-love is not saying yes to others when it means saying no to yourself or, worse, sabotaging yourself.

Lesson: Self-care and preservation are not egomaniacal or selfish traits.

I used to say yes so often when I didn't want to that I would find myself in tears and furious — with no one to blame but myself. If you, too, have a hard time saying no, then you can relate. But the thing is, by saying no to some things you are saying yes to loving yourself. I've been to so many events when I really would have rather been home in my pajamas. The more you say yes to others when you don't want to, the more you ignore your happiness to the point that it affects your health. I realize now that being this way comes from a place of insecurity and trying to strengthen my feelings about myself. I try to escape others' judgment of me. Although compassion and generosity are positive attributes, some-times mine come from this insecure place inside of me, which means I'm giving to get, which is taking a toll on me in the end. This is why the anger resides in me. This is stress on my body. This is Ps on my skin. I had this huge epiphany around the holidays last year and knew I had to love myself more and exercise my "no" muscle. I did, and I must say it felt all too good. If I feared letting someone down, I just knew I had to not care. Obviously, we have to pick and choose our RSVPs, but I felt something incredible lift as I started to say no more in order to spend time with myself.

I'll tell you a secret: If you love yourself enough and do things you love, I assure you more people will be drawn to you and have fulfilling energy versus draining energy. Oddly, instead of wanting to say no, you are going to be dying to do everything they are! Learning to care for yourself is not self-ish. The act of saying no is an act of self-love, so try it and see how your life can change.

Self-love is not being too busy for what's important–YOU!

Lesson: You have value, you are important, just as important as the next person, and you are allowed to be loved in the highest sense by all.

We think we don't have time. We think we have to please everyone else first. I'm very guilty of that. I had horrific time management skills up until this year. My excuse was always "I'm too busy," but somewhere along the way I was so stressed out that I knew if I didn't make time to cook, exercise, relax, and just be, I would live a long miserable life and be covered in Ps. A lot of our days are filled with stress of some kind. My big question for you is: Do you think you can borrow sixty seconds of that time to think of something for which you are grateful? It's that simple! We have time to think about our to-do list, our work, all we need to do at home, our families, etc. That list always continues to grow. If we have time to think and stress about all those things, I think we can borrow sixty seconds from those concerns to sit back and be present for a moment. If you are at work, stop for one minute and listen to the birds outside your window. If you don't have a win-dow, just take some deep breaths, then return to your pile. Stopping for a minute to think of something you're grateful for is a great way mentally to take a break from any stress and become present. It'll also put a smile on your face. Whatever you do for sixty seconds is up to you. Why not have a few ideas in your back pocket and start integrating them into your day? I hope you remember to find gratitude every day, because it will change your life. You just have to focus on ways to take care of yourself. When will it be about you? You are the most important person on this planet and need to love *you*. By doing so, you will be healed, and others will be drawn to giving you the highest love you deserve.

I could go on and on with examples of what self-love is not and lessons that I have learned, but I want to share one more thing with you. It took me a long time to even feel comfortable enough to talk about self-love. It seems so "out there," but somehow, once I got the hang of it, what it involved and what it meant, it became so clear, and now I know how much value was trapped in these two words.

I started by sharing that I had realized that without self-love, nutrition cannot heal you, because you need to love yourself to even eat healthfully. It all starts from there. We are always on this journey; it's like an emotional roller coaster. What comes easily to me now took me five years: the saying no, the fear of judgment, the awkwardness at social outings and not drinking, spending more money to buy healthier food, forcing myself to meditate when all I wanted to do was something else, focusing on changing my negative thoughts, etc. The list can go on and on and believe me, I still have my struggles, too. It's a part of this journey called life!

While on this roller coaster, what does it mean to love yourself? Every time I say to people, "I am a health coach and specialize in helping people with skin disease heal through nutrition and self-love," they look at me funny. They understand the nutrition part, to eat healthier, but they don't understand the self-love part. I don't blame them. After all, I just learned the importance of it myself not too long ago. I'm still figuring out how to explain it, day by day. I have realized that there are all sorts of ways to love yourself but to find them, one must let go. Let go of judgment, let go of where you feel you should be, and let go of all of the berating you do to yourself on a daily basis.

How I started to let go was slowly replacing those thoughts with ones of love. During times of negative thinking, I would consciously make it a point to think thoughts like, "I'm doing the best I can," or "I am healing," or "I am right where I'm supposed to be." It's not easy, by any means. You have to live more in the present moment, and that's tough to do. Once I made the decision to stick to this, it improved my life. I look at things a bit differently now: I see more beauty, take in more awesome moments, and appreciate more of the little things. Imagine how different your life would be if every time you saw your skin disease you thought to give it love instead of hatred. Over time, this became more habitual, and my life is in a very different place now because of it, a much more loving and accepting place.

I find many people are so fixated on the end result in life, not where they are today. Life is too short not to focus on the today. Maybe you work your tail off to get the kids through school, buy the house, the boat, and look forward to retiring when you feel you can finally live and relax. Life is not in the future; it's right now. Self-love is right now. So what can you do for yourself to live and relax right now? This took me years to learn, and I still struggle with it. I worked my butt off in TV production the first eight years of my career, because that's what you do when you get into TV—you work hard. There's no time for self-love, let alone time to call your mother for five minutes! My body broke down, I got sick, I felt miserable and exhausted. Everyone has their boundaries, and I overstepped mine big time.

Without knowing it, I started to love myself more when I decided to pursue my dream to act, which changed my life for the better as well. It made me look deeper inside for answers to find my happiness. Acting made me euphoric for a long time. I've learned that certain opportunities and paths will come into our life to bring us closer to finding our joy. Acting was one of those things for me. It was very therapeutic and forced me to release a lot of emotions I had built up from my past. It was thrilling and fueled my passion. In my experience, when you decide to love yourself to heal, you must feel your pain, your past, and have a conversation with yourself about your issues and what emotions you might be holding on to deep down inside that need to be released and felt. The key here is not to place blame on others for making you feel these emotions, but just own them and sit with them in awareness. Pay attention to your inner dialogue and examine whether it's working for you. Look at your life. Do you complain a lot? Do you automatically think negative thoughts? Take the time to reflect on these things. I know people who think they are very positive, and they will say, "Well, I'm a very positive person." But all I hear are complaints or negative expectations they have about life.

There's a lack of awareness out there, and I believe it stems from a fear of looking at our flaws. What would happen if we started to accept ourselves as we are and owned our flaws or issues as they are, and took responsibility for them? Can you imagine how open this world would be and how healing that could be for us? People would, in turn, be more loving to themselves and one another, because they wouldn't be hiding anything or lying to themselves. I used to lie a lot to myself, which I've learned is the opposite of self-love. You can't love yourself and lie about who you are. You just can't.

Here are a few ways you can love yourself that have changed my life for the better:

- Take things off your plate when you feel overwhelmed.
- Say no to things you don't have time for.
- Treat yourself to a massage.
- Feed your body healthy foods that nourish you.
- Don't work so hard.
- Find ways to lower your stress levels such as with exercise and meditation.
- Participate in activities that are fun.
- Surround yourself with positive, warm-hearted people.
- Work on your relationships to make them strong and healthy.
- Communicate more to let people know what makes you feel good and what doesn't.
- Find ways to enjoy your life outside of work.
- Find ways to enjoy your work.
- Take time to be alone with yourself—whether it's going for a walk or reading a book, get comfortable with you.
- Watch a funny movie.
- Smile more.
- Speak lovingly to yourself. It feels strange in the beginning, but after you do it for a while, your days don't feel the same without hearing those loving words.
- Think about a few things you are grateful for every day.

I think you understand where I am going with this. Do what makes you feel good. Why do we do things at all in this life? We do things because we think we will find happiness in doing them. What makes you happy? Sit and think about that question. Write down a list of things that make you happy. Tuck it away in your wallet and pull it out every once in a while. I guarantee it'll make you smile!

I have a morning routine that has made a difference in my life that I want to share: I wake up and meditate for ten minutes; I make a nice hot mug of water with freshly squeezed lemon and sometimes a little piece of ginger; I sip it while getting ready for my day; while applying coconut oil to my skin, I talk to it with loving words, saying things like, "thank you for working so hard for me," or "I love you and am so grateful you are healing." I'm sure most people hear this and think I'm crazy to talk to my legs, but it feels good. On some level, my body is receiving love, which I believe will help in the healing process. Try it! Think about it for a second, what would help you heal more and enforce all the good things you want in your life—repeating positive affirmations of love, or criticisms that always involve negative thinking?

I also look in the mirror and tell myself I love me almost every day. Sometimes I forget, but I remember at some point. Who else is going to do that every single morning? Okay, well maybe your partner might, but it's not the same thing. It's not coming from inside of you. I learned this mirror exercise from Louise Hay, the bestselling author, speaker and inspirational teacher who has helped thousands of people all over the world. Her books about healing are incredible. I would encourage you to check out *You Can Heal Your Life*. Louise believes a lot of what we say and think tends to be negative and that those words don't create a good experience for us. On her website, she says "A positive affirmation opens the door. It's a beginning point on the path to change. In essence, you are saying to your subconscious mind, 'I am taking responsibility. I am aware that there is something I can do to change.'"[32] When you pay attention to your thoughts, you can begin to eliminate the ones creating experiences you do not want in your life.

Every time I repeat "I love you" to myself in the mirror, I am reminding myself that I'm there for myself in all aspects. I believe that receiving love from myself helps me heal. Without love from ourselves, nothing else can change—not your eating habits, not your weight, not your relationship issues, not your exercise excuses, not your unfulfilling job, not your happiness in life…nothing. Nothing can change unless you start by making a pact with yourself to take better care of yourself—mentally, emotionally, and physically. The biggest lesson I've learned about loving myself is to be my authentic self and to stop hiding parts of me from the world. I suggest you try it; it's incredibly freeing.

Just like the day I wrote about in the previous chapter, where I asked myself: What if this skin condition is from all my anger built up inside of me? What if it never had anything to do with that I ate? What if I created it? If that's the case, I would like to take responsibility for it as well as do something about it. But how? After pondering that question, I finally came to the realization that by loving myself more every day and not being so hard on myself and so critical, that I could move into a better place in life overall.

The key in so many ways is as simple as making the decision to love and honor yourself and your being. For me, it was like a light that came on and I made a decision to put myself

---

32   Louise Hay, "Mirror, Mirror, on the Wall," Heal Your Life blog: http://www.healyour-life.com/mirror-mirror-on-the-wall.

first. Tell yourself, "Now is the time. I'm making a decision to put myself first! Loving myself is now my top priority. Loving me now comes before my family, friends, and even my husband!" Sounds selfish, but it's a good selfish. How can I give all the potential I have to give to others without giving to me first? How can anyone do that? Wouldn't they be doing such a disservice to themselves? The big question is: How do I love myself more? Why does it feel so hard? I think we've been conditioned by our egos and society to beat ourselves up and focus on our shortcomings and failures, rather than on accomplishments and loving moments! All it takes is twenty-seven days of doing something to make it a habit, so what if everyone told themselves they love themselves every day for twenty-seven days? What would happen in their lives?

When I first started on this health journey, I was convinced the message I wanted to spread to the world was about nutrition and how nutrition heals skin disease. Today, I realize and am blown away by the fact that I thought nutrition was just food! I was convinced if I ate well I'd be healthy and Ps-free. I didn't know how much nutrition is actually anything and everything we do to nourish ourselves. And even though my niche is helping people with skin issues, it doesn't matter what illness or condition you have. Everything I teach here can apply to all dis-ease. Loving you, finding happiness in all you do, healthy eating, etc., can help everyone—from people with acne all the way to people with cancer. Nutrition through food was always just a small piece of the big picture. We have to nourish our bodies and our minds, and it's so much more than just what we eat!

When I look back at my life, there I was; I made this change with my food, I was exercising, and I was in a relationship with an amazing man whom I ended up marrying. Things seemed to be falling into place, and I thought I was doing very well for myself, but I wasn't 100 percent happy. Something was missing, and I couldn't figure out what it was. Then it was so clear I couldn't ignore it: I didn't love my job. I was working in TV as a production accountant, and I didn't love it anymore. I wanted to do the acting full time, but that wasn't happening for me. I wanted to give something to the world. I wanted to make a difference. Once I realized I wanted to make a career out of helping people heal their skin, I lit up inside. Everything inside of me was beaming with joy at the mere thought of it. I knew in my bones this was what I was meant to do. Now I've launched my business, written a book, and am helping tons of people! My point in telling you all of this is that now I see the big picture. We need to love ourselves enough to know what we deserve, and love ourselves enough to pursue our dreams. If one part of our lives is unbalanced, we cannot be our happiest and healthiest. We need to find balance in all parts of ourselves.

You have now learned that my struggle has not been an easy or quick one, but I have been successful at healing, and others that have stuck to these principles have been successful, too. So with a little commitment and a lot of this "special" key to unlock the rest of the picture, once you have started to face your emotions, the self-love aspect is the final key that unlocks the door to success. Without it, healing may not transpire on all levels of mind, body and spirit—the levels that we need to become whole, unconditionally loving, and gracious people.

⤜

Ps: Your Ps is the best teacher you've ever had, so honor it and go give it some love. One day it will love you back, cleared and healthy.

Meditation

Study the list at the start of this chapter and then create your own. Think carefully about the ways you sabotage self-love when you're making your list. When you're done, change all the words to what you will do proactively and positively, and work to meditate on them. Repeat them, and when you catch yourself in a negative, say the positive to yourself aloud, because eventually, it will be so. Anything and everything you can do to be a little more loving toward yourself is key.

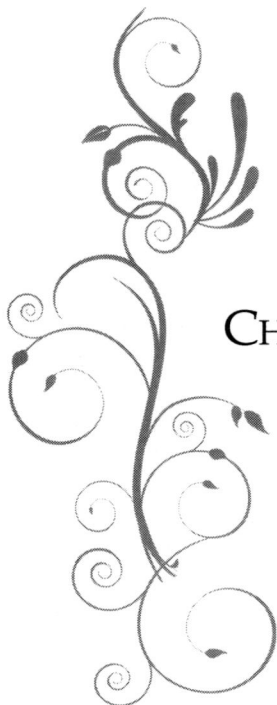

CHAPTER ELEVEN

Practice Makes Perfect: Self-Love, the Holidays and Some Inspiration for You

An ounce of prevention is
worth a pound of cure.

Benjamin Franklin

We have now discussed the importance of self-love and what it means in philosophical terms. So, what does this look like on a calendar or in our daily lives? Let me dive in with what I feel is the hardest holiday first: Christmas. (While I'm going to discuss Christmas, this is really about whatever holiday you celebrate, and maintaining willpower.) I have now learned that to heal, we need to plan and prepare ahead. There are always going to be those days we either love or dread, but so many are composed of the hours and events where people cheat the most every time! I am compiling an inspirational calendar to help you prepare and aid you in your journey of healing, but in the meantime, I hope these blurbs will inspire you to stay strong by preparing ahead.

Holidays and Willpower

I know the holidays are tough for most people, and I didn't prep for them in the early days until after I wrote the blog included below about how the holiday affected me. Re-reading it now, I remain fascinated by human behavior, and I hope you get value from what it says:

The month of December, I had a ton of holiday events and dinners with friends. I was looking forward to all of them, catching up with friends, partying with co-workers, etc. We all know what we look forward to the most: yummy food and alcoholic beverages! The whole "no alcohol" thing was very new to me, and I knew if I didn't plan to fall off the wagon, I'd end up miles from it. I am now giving myself a little credit, considering the holiday season is stressful enough to get through, but I was hanging on to a bit of guilt for sure.

You know: guilt. I learned a long time ago what guilt is: it's sadness or anger from being in a situation you don't want to be in. Well, I'm pretty sure mine was sadness from having this horrible skin disease and anger for having to limit my alcohol intake, even though I'm not a big drinker. I drink so rarely that, when I do go out for drinks, I just want to enjoy one without thinking about its effect on my body. But, this December, I drank about five or six times (and ate yummy, fried, acidic *hors d'oeuvres* several times as well). Not bad, you might say. Well, my skin didn't agree. Soon after, a few little spots appeared, and now I know it was my body telling me it's not okay.

I am experiencing all these emotional gyrations related

to willpower, and somehow I bet I'm not the only one. Having the willpower not to order a glass of wine or not to reach out and grab that delicious-looking appetizer as it passes me was hard. I tried talking to myself: "Kim, it's not worth it, your skin looks amazing, you'll regret it, don't do it!" But that didn't really work. I felt like I had that devil on my shoulder, just like in the movies. The devil was saying, "Screw it! It's the holidays! You can start fresh after the New Year! Have a good time tonight! Get drunk, go on."

It felt tough and, to be perfectly honest, once New Year's passed, I was so glad the holidays were over. I wondered why in the world did I start this new lifestyle in September? Why did I choose to torture myself? I guess I just felt ready at that time. I also realized it all comes down to how you feel, and if you are going to cheat, at least enjoy what you are consuming and say no to guilt. (Again, hard to do!) I found that it didn't feel good to cheat with something like a chocolate chip cookie. If I was going to indulge, I was going for the white chocolate raspberry cheesecake. If I was going to cheat, I was going to make the most of it.

Alcohol and food weren't the only things upsetting my skin. That year, I was feeling a lot of stress. I'm sure you all can relate. The holidays are such a stressful time because you have more on your plate than ever, in a small amount of time. And on top of that, you most likely have to spend a lot of time with people you're not normally around. It all adds up! Stress plays a big part in our body, showing its ugly head in many different ways. I knew I had until the next Thanksgiving to prepare, so I had a little positive chat with myself not to allow the stress, alcohol, or unhealthy food to get under my skin—literally and figuratively!

Being the planner I am, I decided to keep a calendar with positive reminders that I don't need to fall for holiday stress, as well as lots of encouraging ideas in November and December to ensure less stress: take long walks every day; take a bath once a week with Dead Sea salt and lavender oil; spend more time with my pet; get a ten-minute massage from the nail salon once a week (of course now that I live in the 'burbs, I never go); make more time for the extra special family and friends that bring so much love into my life; and make more time for me which is always a constant struggle.

Funny, soon after the New Year, someone special in my life was telling me how rough his holiday was due to stress. He told me something his mom said to him on Christmas that resonated with me. He said that the holiday is just one more day that we get to celebrate being able to live this life, it's no different from any other day. That thought is going to stay with me through every holiday, and I hope you think about that as well.

We all have battles related to a holiday or special event. You just have to try to be ready to make changes in your life, and I hope I have inspired you to find the motivation to experiment so you can figure out what works for you. It's easy to say it, I know, but putting it into action is not so easy. I keep my focus on how I'm feeling, and if I'm feeling good, I know I'm doing something right that my skin will appreciate. Now that I eat 90/10, I can eat healthily almost all the time, and if I really need that piece of cake or those hot wings, well, I can have them. I have found, however, that addressing and preparing ahead of time saves a lot of angst and those feelings of letting yourself down because you were not mentally and physically prepared ahead of time. I hope this helps you think ahead. After all, as I say, "Your skin will love you for this."

Alcohol and Willpower

I can't write a book and not address what every person experiences at some point or another in their life, at a party, an event, or simply getting together with friends: making a decision to use or not use alcohol. The decision is so individual, and I would love to say it won't affect your skin, but it will. How you go about making that personal choice has so many issues attached that I am going to leave that to the brilliant therapists, psychologists, and AA, all of whom know much more than I do on the topic. However, I want to share the act of *not* drinking alcohol and what happens with that, because who knew not drinking could raise eyebrows?

A while back, I had a chat with a friend who has diabetes and gave up alcohol to help himself heal. He was telling me how difficult it was to go out and how he chose to stay in most of the time. My first assumption upon hearing this was that alcohol was just too tempting for him. After all, he used to be a big drinker, and would have a few after work every night. He told me this wasn't the reason, though. It was the way others would react to his not drinking and the way he was treated. He felt like a leper. People looked at him differently and judged him without knowing the why. He said the judgment was so harsh that he was made to feel like something was wrong with him, that he didn't fit in anymore. Some of his friends even stopped contacting him to hang out. He lost a lot of friends because of this. I reminded him those friends didn't deserve him in their life, and he didn't want people like that in his. He agreed, but it didn't make his non-alcohol path easy. It came with a lot of disappointment.

When I decided not to drink anymore during the first year of my journey, I honestly didn't care what anyone thought because I was on to something huge. I was healing my Ps for the first time in almost twenty years! My friends were all incredibly supportive, but over time, I started to notice a few things. Going to happy hour didn't feel as fun, and I didn't feel like I fit in as much as I used to. There was something missing. This was when the mind games began. Also, some of my friends who were so supportive in the beginning started to say things like, "Oh, just have one, it won't kill you," or they would call me "Sober Suzi," or they would egg me on with, "But it's a special occasion!" It started to amaze me how inadequate I felt being in any social position where alcohol was involved. Either my mind games got to me, or my friends' comments did.

I didn't tell my friends how this made me feel. I knew they didn't mean anything malicious by it, nor did they mean to sabotage my health journey. They couldn't relate, and even though they understood the why, they didn't think about how hard I might have been struggling deep down inside. And struggling I was. I would be out for brunch with friends, and watching them have a mimosa started to be hard for me because I wanted one so bad. That had been one of best parts of brunch in the city: good company, unlimited mimosas, a yummy meal, and a great atmosphere. Having a mimosa with brunch reminded me of missing sipping a coffee on my walk to the subway in my morning commute. It was habitual and comforting, and I enjoyed it very much. I almost started to feel like an alcoholic, which I was far from ever being. But not being able to have it made me want it more. You want what you can't have, right?

What kept me motivated was watching my Ps fade away. I knew that mimosa wasn't worth it, and so I continued sipping my herbal tea. Over time, I started to look forward to that tea. Now, I still look forward to that tea, and I don't feel I'm missing out. It brightens my day when I stop to buy a tea on my way somewhere. When my friends are drinking beer and cocktails, I feel happy I'm not putting all that sugar, chemicals, and acidity into my body. I do drink a few times a year, usually on my birthday and on Christmas. I will have whatever I enjoy the most, like a Bellini or a glass of Riesling. My skin doesn't seem to mind too much. It does start to mind when I take advantage of it and drink a few weekends in a row. The more I get to know my body, the more I hear what it is asking of me. I respect and obey it, and in return, it gives me optimum wellness.

I want you to understand that you too might be placed in these odd positions as others react to your lifestyle decisions, and I want to add one last bit about alcohol, because something happened while I was writing this book. Mike and I went out with a few friends, and I noticed this one particular friend of ours who drinks pretty regularly trying to peer pressure me into drinking. I always say no thanks, but she is a bit relentless. Again, I don't think people are being mean when they say things like "You sure, just have one?" or "Oh come on, I'll make you a drink, you'll love it." That night, it hit me (because I had decided to have a drink and she seemed happy and relieved) that *she* isn't comfortable when I don't drink! I'm not sure she even realizes she feels this way.

Mike and I found it fascinating. It's like she can't stand me not drinking because, inside, maybe she feels guilty or self-conscious or something. I don't know what it is, but it was something I thought was interesting: how other people have their issues with alcohol and social situations that may affect you and yours. I'm so fascinated by this because I see clearly how it's so not my issue, it's hers! I always knew that, but I see it now. Something in that behavior makes me feel relieved that it has nothing to do with me.

This doesn't make her a bad person. It just makes her someone I don't want to spend a lot of time with. Her issues force her not to have my best interests at heart. Meanwhile, this is someone who has gone out of her way to cook healthy food for me when I've gone over to her house for dinner. But, I just can't surround myself with people who don't support me one hundred percent, and I encourage you to sit back and look at the people in your life. I know I've driven this point home in other areas of this book, but I want to mention it again. Do the people you spend time with contribute something positive and beautiful to your life? Are they supportive? Are they positive and encouraging and inspiring? I think you get my point. Surround yourself with people who make you feel good about yourself, and don't get peer-pressured into anything. If you choose not to drink, there are many more people out there, these days, who choose the same thing. It's all about you, and all about you making healthy choices for yourself.

Where You Live, Shop, Travel, and Willpower

One of the best things about living in New York City is all the unique and delicious places you can go out to eat. You can go out to a different restaurant every night of the week for five years straight and still have a ton of places to choose from. Having said that, living in NYC with Ps is both easy and hard at the same time. Let me explain by sharing three different experiences I had when eating out with friends in the early days of this journey.

Scenario One:

I went to dinner with friends to celebrate a birthday and had no involvement in picking the restaurant. When this happens, I look up the menu online in advance and see what my options are going to be. I like to be the most prepared when I'm dining out, so I don't need twenty minutes dissecting the menu. After reviewing the small menu, my first thought was "There's nothing I can eat here!" That wasn't actually true; there was one fish dish I could have. So I knew that's what I'd be getting. I was ready to ask the waitress if they could cook it with a little olive oil but was prepared to make an exception if necessary. Fast forward to the actual encounter and the waitress says, "Honey, there's no avoiding butter in this place," I nicely said, "No problem," and I must tell you it was the most delicious piece of fish I've had in a long time. I had forgotten how much butter makes everything taste good! These days, I eat butter sparingly, but I don't need to avoid it altogether like I did at the beginning of my healing journey.

Scenario Two:

I went to visit a dear friend of mine in Brooklyn. He took me to what is the perfect brunch place (for someone without Ps). It was a quaint little place, and I can tell he was excited to take me there. One look at the menu and I honestly didn't know what to do. They had salads, but they were covered in cheese, tomato, peppers, etc. I ended up getting a bed of greens with a side of olive oil and a side of black beans. Out of desperation I also got a side of scrambled eggs (which, at that time, I allowed myself once a week). It wasn't the most enjoyable brunch as I watched my friend inhale his *huevos rancheros*, but luckily the conversation was so good, I wasn't focusing on my bland meal. I count myself lucky that at almost every restaurant in the city you can usually get away with ordering sides, but not at this place, which was a first for me.

Scenario Three:

I planned a brunch date with an old friend and asked her if she'd be willing to try a really good vegan restaurant I had heard of and wanted to try. She was up for it and ended up enjoying it very much. This was a simple experience I wanted to share: great, healthy food and great conversation — simple! These are the types of get-togethers you will start veering toward in your healing journey. It may seem improbable now, but one day, when you step back into that greasy spoon, you will look at the food and go, "No way in heaven am I putting that in my mouth!"

I did learn early with my dietary changes that it felt the easiest when I went food shopping and then cooked in my kitchen, but eating out is an issue we all will face at some time or another. It takes thinking and preparation, which isn't so bad when you get the hang of it. Now I'm a new type of foodie who looks at NYC in a new light and realizes there is a point to living in a city with such diverse and healthy food choices, if you are willing to look.

Again, I just want to say there are a few things I learned having these experiences, and I hope you do too. The first and biggest one is that my health comes before pleasing people. I don't know about you, but this was a tough one for me because I don't want to be that person who comes off like a diva. I also didn't want to be that person who orders a salad on a date, because that's not who I am. I'm a woman with a big appetite, and I love to share the experience of food and dining out.

The hard part is that if you are unprepared and then stressed over a menu, you have already taken the enjoyment out of getting together, so my second point is to prepare as much as you possibly can before eating out. From researching the menu, to throwing nuts or mini-seasonings in your purse for emergencies, you can save awkward, nervous, guilty feelings that are stressful on the body and the mind and just enjoy yourself and your time with others.

Third, find friends who are understanding and supportive.

This is huge. Anyone who doesn't support me in my journey will not be fortunate enough to dine with me anymore. This is about honoring your body and yourself and finding loving, supportive, and nurturing people who will help you heal more quickly. Fighting the negative thoughts, emotions, and reactions of other people only wastes valuable time, and we don't have time for that when we are on a healing journey.

Being Single to Being with Someone and Willpower

Life is all about change and transitions, and you never realize how much is involved until you are knee-deep in it, so I found this little journal section I wanted to share:

Summer has been a little rough. Not terrible, but lately I've found myself lacking the self-control I need for this journey. I think it has a lot to do with being in a relationship. The two of us just have so many plans and things to do. This is not a bad thing, but every single party we go to, or wedding, or day on a boat, or hiking trip is a situation that demands planning. It's a lot of thinking to do. It's so easy and convenient to just not think about it and grab something quick while you are out, but bringing something to the party that you can eat or eating before you go complicates matters.

When I was single, I was the only one to worry about, I guess. I had my routine of places I'd go to grab my veggies before I went home and if I got together with friends, they knew and understood my journey, and we went to restaurants that were vegan/vegetarian-friendly. We still do. It's easy in the city to find a healthier place to eat, but it's a bit tougher out in Long Island where there are mostly just chain restaurants. I've only found one good vegan place to eat, and it's still pretty far from me. There are farmer's markets here and there, which are nice, but I realized, I can get twice as much organic food from Trader Joe's at the same cost. And I love farmer's markets. It's not that I don't want to support them, it's just tough on a budget.

🐚

When I re-read this, I realized that the first time I started this change I was single, and being single and eating as constricted as you want is so much easier. So I want to make sure that I address how those of us in relationships and with families and children do have extra planning to do. The big question, however, is how can we remain strong and not feel the need to do as they do or eat as they eat? Here are a few stories that I do hope you can relate to.

First, I have to admit my life as a single woman living in the city was amazing. I enjoyed being single and only having to worry about myself. There was something very freeing in that, especially when my healing journey began. I was definitely meant to be alone during that time because I spent a lot of it researching, reading, watching documentaries, attending seminars and workshops, etc. I needed to dive into the health world and be a sponge to soak up every bit of information I could about healing. I had my routine of going to the farmer's market across the street from my apartment, getting all my healthy items to juice and cook with, and returning home to prepare my meals. It was pretty easy only thinking about myself. When I would go out to dinner or brunch with friends,

I would ask them if we could go to a vegan restaurant or a place that has a load of healthy options for me to choose from.

Then I met Mike. I admit, I got a little caught up and thrown off track when we first started dating, because I wanted to take him to all sorts of unique places to eat when he would come into the city to visit me. This calmed down after a while, and I would cook very healthy meals for us. But I loved introducing him to all sorts of yummy, spicy, saucy foods he had never tried before, like Indian and Ethiopian. I had to take him to Grimaldi's in Brooklyn. He loves pizza and had never even walked across the Brooklyn Bridge to experience it! (Grimaldi's is right under the bridge.) It's such a romantic date—how could I not take him there? Actually, it was that date when he first said I love you, so, you see? All that acidity, sugar, and dairy worked for me after all! When you eat out you never really know what's in the sauce or the spice. What if it has paprika? (That's a nightshade.) Or sugar in the sauce? (Which causes all sorts of inflammation.) You don't know what oil it's cooked in. Is it butter or canola oil? It's like the day Max's vet told me that dog food is leftover scraps and "you don't know what's in it."

When Mike came along, everything changed. I was now traveling to stay with him on the weekends, and we were going out more with different friends or taking weekend trips. We were busy, and I realized, very quickly, I needed to get back on track, but now with him in my life, it was harder. The first thing I did was have him pick up some things that he could always have on hand in his kitchen when I stayed over. Things like brown rice, veggies, fruit, and herbs and spices like turmeric, cinnamon, tea, and so on. All of my staples that I would want to have to commute to work with a hot beverage in hand, as well as some nourishing foods to eat for dinner for when I returned. It made a difference, and Mike learned to ask me every week what I needed from the store. It was nice that he wanted to take care of me.

We got a groove going and it was a little easier for me, but I was also still living in the city where I could grab a quick bite at a healthy vegan café on my way home if I didn't feel like cooking. It wasn't like this where Mike lived, outside of the city in the suburbs, so it took a lot of effort and planning on the days we'd see each other. I dreamed of the time we'd move in together because I just knew it would make our lives so much easier in the food aspect.

A friend of mine who is married had asked me to think about writing a blog about cooking for two because he was trying to lose weight at the time and wanted to go on a strict diet, but felt bad he wouldn't be eating meals with his wife. I loved this question because it made me think of my internal struggle with it and how our groove took time and effort, but was so worth it. That groove we set into motion three years ago is now easy-peasy living together.

My biggest piece of advice for anyone living together is to come up with some staple dishes that you both like. Sit down and talk about what healthy foods you both enjoy, write up a list, and think of ideas—maybe even Google some easy recipes. Luckily Mike likes what I eat—all sorts of veggie dishes, salmon, sometimes chicken, salads, healthy versions of desserts and snacks, etc. — but he also likes a lot of things I don't allow myself, like beer and pizza.

We have a few meals that have become staples in our kitchen that we both agree are our official go-tos when we are thinking about our big food shop for the week:

- Baked salmon with sautéed broccoli and/or kale.
- Spaghetti squash: I like mine with a little olive oil and sea salt; Mike likes his with tomato sauce and ground turkey.
- Sweet potato fries, baked and sprinkled with cinnamon and nutmeg. Always a good option when craving carbs!
- Our healthy version of chicken and fried brown rice: brown rice, egg, frozen peas and carrots, shredded chicken with olive oil, and liquid aminos.
- Homemade soup: Mostly, in the winter, we'll make a big pot of homemade chicken soup with quinoa/ brown rice noodles. I've also made butternut squash, apple, carrot soup and Peruvian quinoa soup, which is our new favorite. We'll also make a stew in the crock pot with all sorts of veggies and organic chicken. These dishes are good because they will last a few days.
- Salads: I try to vary it up with different greens, shredded carrots, cucumber, chickpeas, (a little shredded parmesan cheese for Mike), and a vinaigrette I whip up with fresh lemon juice, olive oil, apple cider vinegar, garlic, salt, and pepper.

When I am not home, Mike has his staples:
- Pizza
- Turkey burger
- Tacos with ground turkey

His staples may not be as healthy as our shared list, but we can't completely deprive ourselves, either. It's that 90/10 lifestyle.

Sometimes we find ourselves sitting together eating two completely separate meals, but hey, as long as we are both happy, who cares? I might crave a bowl of brown rice/quinoa pasta with sautéed broccoli, and he might make himself a turkey burger. Either way, I always have these items in the house: veggies, fruit, organic eggs, organic chicken, wild-caught salmon, sweet potatoes, various grains, brown rice/quinoa pasta, beans, nuts, seeds, Ezekiel sprouted bread, and almond butter. Mike has all of that plus his personal favorites like turkey burgers, cheese, cold cuts, and sourdough bread. He has happily been lowering his cheese intake as well as experimenting with lunches besides cold cuts. I'm happy to have had this positive influence on him. One day, I might even get him off the nitrates.

All in all, find your groove by finding the foods you both like and together create some staple dishes. Those staple dishes saved us some major stress. Especially since I used to not get home from work until 8:00 p.m. and I didn't want to have to think about cooking starting that late. The plan had to be made ahead of time. Otherwise, we'd be eating at 10:00 p.m. every night.

I always wished I had more time to experiment with different recipes, but that's what the weekends are for. I advise you to get your family and friends on board. It's so much easier on this path when you have support. I'm learning to do the best I can, because that really is enough! The key is this: communicate, plan, and make the effort together. Your relationship will grow stronger because of it. But, if your partner is not ready for that journey, then just quietly do it for yourself because it is amazing how our actions and our vibrant health speak louder than words.

And now for some inspiring thoughts and suggestions of how to make it through the hard times because I don't want you to forget to give yourself self-love during all these stressful events. Here's a blog post I did about self-love during the holidays—because as long as we are alive, there will be another one of them to conquer!

Self-love This Holiday Season[33]

The holidays are stressful. With shopping, attending parties, wrapping up things at work, and preparing for the new year, there's no end of things on the calendar. This season, I am feeling that stress more than ever, and it's forcing me to look at myself very deeply. It's hard to squeeze in any me-time in December, and I always look forward to my break from work because it's a week where I can make a few dates with myself and catch up on my life without feeling like I have to squeeze it in.

I didn't realize how much me-time I needed until recently when I had a bit of a meltdown that brought me to tears. The truth is, I haven't been making myself a priority these past few months, and I'm feeling all sorts of guilt and anger with myself. Filling up my calendar is no one's fault but my own. I know this. So why do I constantly do it during a time when I need to have space and time to myself more than usual?

I dug deep within myself to understand why this is such a struggle, and why it's so hard for me to say no. This is what I learned: I love the people in my life so much, and they bring me so much love. I want to see

---

33 https://healingmypsoriasis.wordpress.com/2015/12/18/self-love-this-holiday-season/ (originally posted December 18, 2015).

them and spend quality time with all of them—I genuinely do. The issue is that, between a busy work schedule, attending school, and taking care of myself, there isn't a lot of time left. Life is busy, isn't it?

So why can't I say no? Don't get me wrong, I do say no all the time. But I say yes more times than I want to. Part of me does so because I genuinely want to see my friends and family. The other part is because I have a deep need to please people. I can't tell you the uncomfortable emotions that come up in me when I admit that, but it's 100 percent true—and I want to start standing in my truth more. I do a disservice to myself when I don't.

While being a people pleaser and a bit of a perfectionist might sound like positives, those are two things that will stand in your way to living a truly happy life. One thing I've learned through years of therapy is that you cannot be truly happy while needing to be in control. It's just not possible, even if we convince ourselves otherwise. I've worked very hard on my issues over the years, but they still pop up here and there. When they do, I always think, "Really? Are you still here? I thought I got rid of you!"

I am learning that just because we are aware of our issues and work on them doesn't mean they just disappear. I think they stay with us on some subconscious level to remind us of the lessons we are here to learn. For me, that lesson is about self-care and love. I need to practice a lot of it in this lifetime to live my happiest.

That means saying no more often to everyone else and saying yes more often to me.

To that end, I've added a few small, loving things I've incorporated into my mornings to give myself a little love on a daily basis, which I've listed below. If these resonate with you on some level, in any aspect of your life, maybe they can help you too:

- **I meditate for ten minutes**: Every morning is different. Sometimes I lie in bed and sometimes I do it on the train on my way to work. I plug in my earbuds and listen to soothing music. I breathe and pay attention to it. Every time a thought pops into my head, which is about every 5-10 seconds, I ask it to leave and return my attention to my breathing and silently repeat "let go" or "release."
- **I boil water and squeeze fresh lemon into it with a slice of ginger**: I sip it while getting ready in the morning. It's detoxing, energizing, and warming to my soul. It also cleans me out … if you know what I mean.
- **I massage my skin with coconut oil**: I massage it with grateful thoughts, knowing its healing properties are giving my skin much-needed love.
- **I talk to my skin and tell it how much I appreciate and love it**: It needs love too, you know! After all, it's our largest organ and has a lot of work to do every day!
- **I look in the mirror, look into my eyes, and say "I love you" three times**: This might sound strange, but we need love every day and what better way to give it to ourselves? As strange as it feels at first, I guarantee it will eventually make you smile.

Before we move on to our final Ps and meditation, I want to share another blog with you that I wrote. I want you to keep these ideas in your head every day if you can, and every moment when you are feeling a little off or confused, because healing comes when you are present with yourself and able to say YES! to life and healing:

Be Present Enough to Say YES! to Life[34]

I was sitting in my kitchen eating lunch, trying to be present with my food, when I noticed a huge part of me wanted so badly to bring it back to my desk and eat while I worked. I actually grabbed my bowl and proceeded to get up until I caught myself. I stopped, sat down, put my food back on the table, and thought, "Whoa, what was that? My computer and phone can wait! I'm going to eat my lunch and be with my food now."

So I took a few bites, tried to focus on the taste and chewing, but it felt really hard to stay put. Everything in me wanted to get work done while I ate. Everything! I even giggled a little because I couldn't believe I felt that out of control. Why in the world couldn't I just sit there for ten minutes and enjoy my meal? What was so pressing? The answer is nothing. But my mind didn't think so. I realized, at that moment, by staying put I was saying "no" to say "yes" to myself—saying "yes" to being more present, as hard as it felt at that moment.

I've been thinking about saying yes more to life in ways that I haven't been, such as being present with my food

---

34   https://healingmypsoriasis.wordpress.com/2016/01/15/being-present-enough-to-say-yes-to-life/ (January 15, 2016).

when I eat. This made me think about an event I attended back in the fall. It was Kris Carr's new book launch, where she talked all about saying yes to life. It was an amazing event, and I was so excited I finally got to meet her because she is my biggest role model! It was her and two other incredible ladies, Gabrielle Bernstein and Marie Forleo, who changed my life. (If you are unfamiliar with these three inspirational women, I urge you to Google them.)

Kris opened up the night by sharing an "Aha!" moment she had. She was working on the new book and was feeling uninspired and exhausted. While venting to her husband, he said, "Let's just go do something fun. Let's get out of here." Kris did something she wouldn't normally do when she has a deadline; she went with him for a bike ride in the woods. As she was riding, she stopped to look up, feeling a bit overwhelmed by all of the beauty—the colorful trees, birds singing, various sounds of plant and animal life, etc.—and said she found herself sitting in mother nature thinking, "YES!" She felt invigorated at that moment and thought about how beautiful and amazing life is. Right then, she was inspired and felt open to everything.

Kris jokes about saying no all the time and how she likes to be at home all comfy in her pajamas, so the next time she received an invitation to a party, she said yes—all because of her experience in the woods that day. She went and ended up meeting someone who invited her to an event where he was giving a talk. Again, she would normally have said no, but she felt compelled to say yes, and as she walked into this event, she noticed a poster for it that stated the topic of the talk, which was "Saying Yes to Life."

Something on that bike ride told her to say yes to life, and she heard it loud and clear. She was amazed at how the universe spoke to and guided her toward more happiness and fulfillment. She wanted to share this story to remind us to listen and say yes more.

Do you ever find yourself having one of those moments where you feel so damn inspired and excited and scared (a good scared)? Maybe something wonderful just happened in your job, or you met someone, or maybe you are just going for a run or a bike ride, like Kris, and feel something great inside of you for no reason. Maybe something is just reminding you of how beautiful and perfect you are, and you feel it throughout your entire body. I think we all have these awesome moments. They might feel rare, but they come more often when you are open for them. I try my best to be present so that, when they come, I'm ready, willing, and able to say yes to them.

Synchronicity is what happened to Kris when she went for that ride in the woods, and she was present enough to hear and feel it. My teacher, Joshua Rosenthal, at the Institute for Integrative Nutrition, says that once we develop a knack for noticing and welcoming synchronicity, life becomes more interesting and rewarding. We start to meet the right people at the right time to lead us to the next station in life.

I try my best to be present enough to read the signs and feel the direction my life wants to go. This reminds me of birds when they fly together. I have recently gotten into watching and admiring the synchronicity of them as they fly overhead in big waves, and not one is out of alignment. I think it's the coolest thing! To me, it's a huge sign that there is something bigger happening here beyond just us.

One morning, I was standing on the train platform with a ton of other commuters, waiting for our train to arrive. I was watching in awe as the birds circled above our heads. I swear they knew I was watching and were saying something to me! Maybe they were saying good morning! So I said (to myself), "Morning, birdies!"

I glanced over at the pack of people huddled where the train doors usually stop. No one was looking at the birds. Not one person. Instead, they were all looking down and appeared quite tired, cranky and unhappy. I looked at all these people all around me, and then back up at the large flock of birds circling so gracefully over our heads, round and round. The birds just didn't stop, and it was so obvious they were trying to get our attention! I was mesmerized, and couldn't believe no one else was even looking. They were going to miss them completely in thirty seconds! I wanted to shout, "Wake up, people!"

Many of us miss the beauty of the everyday. That used to be me. I was so busy, consumed by my job, working countless hours, caring too much what others thought, and covering up my skin, that I missed all the beauty around me. It took a while, but I have finally arrived and am the most awake I've ever been. I love this beautiful life! I love that I have this skin disease, because it has changed my world for the better and woke my ass up! I love that it helped teach me to become more present than I've ever been my whole life.

When we are present, we are saying YES! to life. Next time you are outside, look for the birds. They will appear. And when they do, I bet you'll never miss them again.

Back in my kitchen, I wrote this blog in my mind as I ate my lunch. Then I heard my phone beeping. Someone was texting me! I smiled, wanting so badly to see who it was. Instead, I sat there and finished my lunch.

I hope you all also have the most beautiful, synchronistic moments in the New Year!

Ps: Be still. Ask your body what it needs to heal and watch the answers start coming to you. Have it tell you what an ideal calendar, an ideal life looks like. In your heart, you know the answers, so it is a matter of loving yourself enough to complete the follow-through and be present.

🕮

Meditation

There will always be stuff we need to do, people we need to see, foods we need to eat, obligations we need to fill, and work we need to finish. We will never really get it all done, will we? It will always keep on coming. Let your new goal be to work toward being present, living in the now moment because that's really all we have, isn't it? Right now. Not the past, not the future, only now!

And I want to interject here that there is never an ideal time to start a healing journey, because some event is always around the corner, so just dive in and start today. The time is now.

And in the now, we have a choice of focusing on the positive or negative, and if our focus on the positive makes us feel good, then why focus on anything else? Why please others who may not have your best interest in mind?

As a meditation, pick one of these five ways to get you out of your head and into the present and try doing one of these, every day!

1. Before you drift off to sleep, think of two things you are grateful for.
2. Leave your phone at home and take a walk around the block. Take in the trees, grass, sounds, etc.
3. Stop what you're doing and take three deep breaths, paying attention only to your breathing.
4. Take in the synchronicity of the birds, next time you have the opportunity.
5. Say "I love you" to yourself in the mirror while you get ready in the morning.

Make it a priority today to calm your mind, even if just for one minute. Pay attention to anything besides your thoughts and you will witness your life change before you. In this exercise, do something spiritual (whatever that is for you, it doesn't have to be meditation), do affirmations, say loving things to yourself, pay attention to nature, be present, focus rather than being on autopilot, follow your passion or at least do stuff that you enjoy, surround yourself with healthy friends and family, cleanse toxic people from your life, keep a journal or a vision board, make a gratitude list, visualize, pray. Do whatever you need to do, but don't forget to say YES! to life.

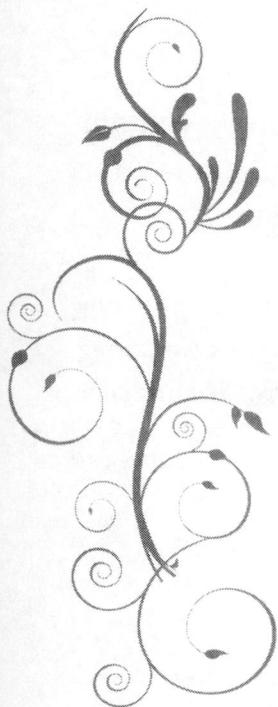

In Conclusion

*Nobody grows old by merely
living a number of years.
We grow old by deserting our
ideals. Years may wrinkle the
skin, but to give up enthusiasm
wrinkles the soul.*

Samuel Ullman

From the bottom of my heart, I want to thank you for saying yes to life and for taking this journey with me. Somehow, in writing this book, I have exposed even deeper parts of myself than I had ever guessed were ready to come out. I do believe that enthusiasm and passion are what make us truly alive, and if I had not been chosen to suffer from this horrible *dis-ease*, I would not have been called to help and heal others. A dear friend of mine once said, "Nurturing and growing, when met with unconditional love, equals miracles." Nothing can stop you when the love you show yourself and then to others overrides the past emotions you harbored. My love is so deep for your healing process and success, I put it all out there. Join me in the revolution for health, for feeling settled and loving your skin, to continual healing and spreading of unconditional joy. Contact me, email me, reach out; your time for change is now.

Our body is precious.
It is our vehicle for awakening.
Treat it with care.

Buddha

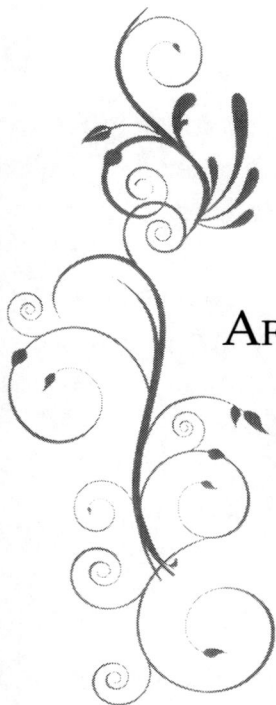

My Personal Journey: Who Am I to Give Advice? After All, I'm Not a Doctor

I have pretty thick skin,
and I think if you're going to be
in this business, if you're going
to be an actor or a writer,
you better have a thick skin.

John Irving

As much as I have written this book to share my personal story, I have left some of the details about myself until the end. I wanted to make this book as useful as possible to readers up front, and if you needed to hear my personal story, here you go!

I grew up in Long Island, New York, and had what feels like a pretty normal childhood despite the effects of a dysfunctional family life: my father was an alcoholic, and my mother had a few bouts of crazy because of it. Let me just say this: the woman knows how to throw a dish! But despite all the screaming and fighting that went on, I went to church every Sunday, played kickball outside with my neighborhood friends, grew up to have a successful career in TV and film, and have had a pretty busy social life with loving friends. Luckily, I started working on my unresolved issues in therapy during my teenage years — and there were a bundle. I found myself aware enough to return to therapy in my twenties and again in my thirties when needed. I encourage everyone to seek out a good coach, mentor, or therapist.

I am the youngest of three girls, and I take after my dad, a very loving and giving personality — to a fault sometimes. I believe very much in love conquering all and am extremely good at giving it to others. I'm finally working on giving it to myself, which was really tough at first.

I developed psoriasis at nineteen. I actually can't seem to remember exactly when I saw it for the first time. What seems to really stick out in my mind was when I was twenty-one and in Cancun, Mexico on spring break with a group of friends. We were hanging out by the pool, and my legs were covered in these small, red, scaly spots. The sun was blazing, and the spots were lobster red. A few of my friends were asking what that was all over my legs, and I was mortified. I managed to act as if it wasn't a big deal and would quickly jump in the pool. Meanwhile, inside I was *dying* of embarrassment! At that age, all I cared about was what people thought. All my female friends were feeling so good in their skin, so confident. I was beyond self-conscious and spent the week thinking about why this *dis-ease* chose me, why this exact moment in time, and why had it come to ruin my life. My trip was ruined by all of my negative thinking, and I'm sure my negative thoughts only brought on more spots. It didn't help that I had a huge crush on one of the guys we were with, who I'm sure could sense my insecurity from miles away.

After this trip, I went to see a dermatologist. As I mentioned in Chapter Two, I tried what the medical doctors told me to do. I applied steroid creams and constantly had to change them up over the years. They certainly helped at times. Tanning helped too, but it's expensive, and deep down I knew it wasn't good for me. (Tanning salons are banned in some countries due to the cancer link and it's still a hot topic of discussion in America.) I came very close to getting laser treatments, but they were too costly and too time-consuming.

Most people in my life didn't even know I had Ps because I covered it up so well over the years, and if I had a breakout I was all over it, doing whatever it took — new creams, tanning, Revlon cover-up — you name it. Anything to not feel at its mercy!

During those formative years, all I ever wanted to do was act. I performed in all my high school plays and couldn't wait to get out there into the real world and chase my dream. The day came when I was applying to get into Marymount Manhattan College (MMC) and my two subject choices were to major in acting or theater history. I chose theater history. Why? Because I was terrified. I didn't have enough confidence. It was not just my Ps, but it certainly didn't help make me feel good or good enough to get on a stage and have all attention on me.

I graduated from college, did well in classes, and had lots of friends, yet I was full of the fear of being judged. So, I chose theater history and put my acting dream behind me. I had a wonderful experience at MMC, met some like-minded people, got a good education, and looked forward to a career behind the scenes. Of course, deep inside, I wanted to be on that stage. I can now see I repressed any and all feelings during my time in college.

I grew my career in TV and film behind the scenes, working in production management for six years. During that time and despite my fears, I started acting when I was thirty. To give myself more flexibility, I switched from production management to production accounting, and went out hustling, hitting the ground, running, trying to book auditions and jobs every day.

I cannot tell you the fear that would creep in being an actress with Ps. The thought was always somewhere hidden in my brain, "I will be mortified if the wardrobe doesn't cover up my Ps." I would have an audition, and if the film took place in the summer—where I'd be expected to be wearing shorts or there was an indoor scene at night where I'd be wearing a nightgown—in the back of my mind, the thought was always there that my secret would be exposed. I was constantly guessing. *What will the director think? Will they be understanding or will they be disgusted and think it is contagious?* In my mind, I would inevitably be fired from that role.

At that time, it didn't even dawn on me that Ps was not what I should really be focusing on. I should be focusing on doing a good job, getting into the character, playing with it, and most of all, having fun doing what I love. Believe you me, I know we are in control of how we live our life, whether we choose happiness or not, but Ps has this way of seeping into every part of your life, and because it's on the outside for everyone to see, it's extremely difficult to not care what others think. It makes you feel ugly and ashamed. I don't know anyone with this disease who doesn't care what others think.

I went on trying to live my life, trying to be a success, trying to pretend that the thing I feared most on my skin was not there and all my time was focused on not letting others see it. I lived my life in hiding, constantly covering up, and only after healing myself did I realize that feeling of freedom was foreign to me. It felt like nothing I've ever felt—simply amazing. To not have something looming over you, nothing extra for your mind to dwell on, think about, figure out every moment of every day is incredibly freeing. It was like I could breathe again!

When I healed my Ps the first time around, I felt what it was like not to care anymore. It felt like ease. Can you imagine going about your life with ease and flow, not allowing every thought to be about hiding your skin? It was an incredible feeling.

We all have different careers, some where you don't need to worry about what you are going to wear, and some where you do. My day job requires me to dress casually, which enables me to cover up my sensitive areas. I'm lucky. But with my acting, I didn't have a choice what I wore if I was cast in a role. It was a very scary feeling, but no way did it stop me from chasing my dream, and I hope it doesn't stop you!

I may have had these negative thoughts with the fear of being "found out," but I wanted so badly to act that if it came with embarrassing moments, so be it. If anything, the acting and my fear of people seeing my Ps have had a huge impact on my effort toward my healing journey.

Not only was I silently struggling with Ps but all the way into my late teens, I had yet another secret. My father was an alcoholic, and I did everything I could to protect and hide it from others. When successful, I would have a moment of feeling in control.

Growing up in an alcoholic home contributed to my fair share of issues, all of which I realize now manifested Ps in some ways. A child that grows up in a chaotic, unstable, unsafe, uncontrollable world often carries over the biggest issue: that of needing to be in control.

Here is an example of what I remember. (My mom would tell this story differently, but my sister and I remember the incident the same way and it has always stuck with us.) It's the one memory from childhood that comes up again and again for me. One day my parents got into a horrific fight, glasses and dishes were broken. Because I was the baby, my sisters tried to protect me by locking me away in their room upstairs. In a desperate attempt to fix the situation (keep in mind I was five), I ran to the top of the staircase where I could see them, stuck my head through the tiny banisters, and screamed for them to stop. To my complete surprise, I suddenly realized my head was stuck, and there was no way out. Fortunately, this predicament stopped the fighting, because now they had a bigger problem! The neighbor ended up getting me unstuck with his hacksaw, and I came out unscathed—at least physically.

We all have these stories to some degree, but looking back now I realize how I would do anything to break up these arguments or try to be the peacekeeper, all as a way to control my environment and the people in it.

My control issues grew worse in my young teenage days when controlling anything made me feel safe in the chaotic environment of my house. That's when I became more and more committed to cleaning. I used to clean up after my dad all the time, and I realize now it was to hide the evidence. When my friends would come over, I'd feel embarrassed if the house was messy or dirty, so I would always clean up. I think I just didn't want them to know he drank. If he left a dish in the sink, I'd clean it. If he left a ring on the counter from his cup, I'd clean it. You name it, I'd clean it.

I grew up wanting to feel safe in what felt like an unsafe environment, so I would clean up after *everyone*, try to fix *everything*, and try to show the world how happy I was. I'm not sure, looking back, if this was something I did more for me or others, but it led to me becoming a bit of a perfectionist, as well as a people pleaser. While these might sound like positive traits, they are two things that will stand in your way to living a truly happy life. I developed a reputation in my family for being a control or clean freak. My sisters sure did appreciate it, though, once they moved out and needed me to clean their new house or apartment!

I know my parents did the best they could. I truly mean that. People do the best they can, considering how they were raised and what their issues might be. My dad was an alcoholic, and he did the best he could at that time. His addiction drove my mom crazy because she wanted to rely on him, and she probably wanted to feel just as safe as we wanted to. As I write this, I can hear the voice of my mom and sisters saying that they can't agree with me. They would say, "He didn't do the best he could. He drank and didn't take care of his family. Why would you say that he did his best?" I understand that view completely. If someone is unemployed and has a family to provide for, you would think they would be knocking on every door and be willing to work for minimum wage or less, just to have a job, right? But sometimes they don't, and their families refer to them as losers without ever really knowing what is going on inside them. Maybe the afflicted individual is filled with fear or has a complete lack of self-worth. I'm just saying you don't really know, and I would like to give my dad credit for being sick at that time—mentally, emotionally, and physically—and I guess that's why I feel he did do his best.

I believe the universe puts us on the path of least resistance to getting what we want, but sometimes it sure as hell doesn't feel like that. It feels hard. But when you fast-forward and look back, you can see how that path steered your life and where it's brought you today. Please, don't get me wrong, a parent that's a falling-down drunk, verbally and physically abusive to their spouse and children, or sexually abusing family members is nowhere near able to try to or be their best and needs to be removed for the safety of the family until the situation can be resolved. This was not my scenario, and I am grateful for that.

What I am saying is that, if I hadn't grown up in an alcoholic home, I would not have some of the issues I've had growing up. If I didn't have those issues, I might not have gotten Ps. If I didn't have Ps, I would never have found my life's calling or be able to help others the way I am today.

I wouldn't take back a single sad moment of my life. As I write this, I'm tearing up thinking of all the innocence I lost at such a young age due to my dad's drinking. I can remember my mom always feeling so helpless and stuck. She, of course, never realized at the time how wrong this was, but she would have my sisters and me look for all of his vodka bottles hidden in the chairs and couches, and while he was sleeping, we'd empty them, fill them with water, and put them back. Supposedly, he never knew!

As I said, my mom did the best she was able to do given her circumstances. Today, we talk about it and she admits she didn't realize that it was wrong back then. I think she was in a very panicked state of mind, not being able to control my dad's drinking while trying to raise the kids and trying to survive herself. Luckily my dad was a very reclusive alcoholic.

He rarely came out of the bedroom, or else he'd just sit in his chair and stare at the TV. I had a friend in high school whose dad was a raging alcoholic and beat her. So compared to her, I was fortunate.

Another odd fact is that I honestly never realized that my dad being an alcoholic was abnormal. I really didn't. There was always this elephant in the room, so to speak, because no one would talk about it, but I didn't realize how different my home environment was until I was in high school and started spending a lot of time at my friends' houses. They would invite me to have dinner with them all the time or to go away with them. My family never ate dinner together. My mom swears we did, but I don't really remember all of us sitting around the table eating as a family, talking about our day. Maybe we did; I don't remember. I'm pretty sure I blocked out a lot of my childhood because I can't really remember much.

I do remember playing ball outside with the neighborhood kids, going to block parties, and things like that. It really felt like a very normal childhood, except a few memories of my mom crying, throwing plates, and sitting on the grass out front of our house, sobbing. My mom doesn't remember doing this, but that remains to be argued. I do remember my dad coming to my middle school once, taking me out of class, and carrying me to the car while I was hysterically crying. The principal was following us, trying to get my dad to let go of me, because my mom had called the school telling them not to allow him to take me out. They thought he was kidnapping me. Turns out, they'd had a bad fight and he wanted me to console him. He needed someone, and that someone was always me.

I was very close to my dad, a total daddy's girl. No matter how much he drank and didn't take care of my mom or us kids, I always felt for him. I saw his pain, and I don't think anyone else in my family saw that. They just saw a man who could not get his act together and support his family. Again, I get it, I really do. I had sympathy for my dad; they were angry.

Things didn't seem to get too hard for me emotionally until high school. I am pretty sure all of the issues I was starting to develop were somewhere hiding in my subconscious and, now in my high school years, they were ready to show themselves. Makes sense, right? In high school it's about finding yourself, fitting in, finding love, etc. I think, all of a sudden, I started becoming more aware, and I'm positive being around functional families opened my eyes a bit. I also started to see a counselor who spoke openly with me about my dad's drinking. That changed everything. I actually wrote her a letter a few years ago thanking her for the difference she made in my life back then. She was very shocked and pleased to get my letter twenty years later.

In high school I wanted everyone to like me. I think that's where my people-pleasing tendencies really hit their stride. I already had control issues, and now I had people-pleasing issues as well. I cared what people thought. I wanted them to see the happiest me, because maybe if they saw that they wouldn't see my pain. I didn't know how to love myself back then. I joke about it now, passing it off as if to say, "Does anyone that age know how to love themselves?"

Looking back, I can see that's all I needed, some love from me. I had wonderful friends, many of whom are still in my life today. I had a boyfriend who didn't really know how to show me love, but this was high school, so I can't hold it against him. It wasn't until my twenties that I realized I had a pretty good personality and was very open and expressive. People liked my energy and it even got me jobs. I was always naturally charismatic and happy. Seriously, my friends would describe me as the most positive and happy person they knew.

I really feel that a happy and positive state of mind is my most natural state. It's not fake and I'm not trying to be dramatic. I'm expressive and loving and warm, and I like to show it. My issue with that is that I don't feel comfortable being anything but happy. So where is my anger, jealousy, resentment, sadness, and all those negative emotions?

That thought of where all those emotions end up is what led me to question if, perhaps, that was what ended up coming out of my skin. I would never complain, or say no, or be angry with anyone, or let anyone see anything negative about me—but why? Because I wanted them *all* to like me. A therapist I used to see once said, "Kim, not everyone is going to like you," and I replied, "But why not?" She said, "That's not possible, and you have to accept that." I remember feeling very uncomfortable with that thought. Funny, I saw that therapist in my twenties when I was finding myself, fitting in, and seeking love in the big city.

Then, as the years went by, something changed, and I changed. Things became so different in my thirties. I found myself. I chose to "fit out" when not fitting in, and I found love. Most importantly, I learned how to give myself love.

The people pleaser in me still struggles with saying no, and I like feeling a sense of control, but those issues are now a bit more resolved after having worked on them so many years. My husband makes fun of me sometimes when we have an insanely busy week, and dishes are left for days in the sink. He'll joke and say, "Honey, you going to be able to sleep tonight with those dishes in the sink?" Cracks me up just thinking about it. He's asking me that not because he's ever witnessed me *needing* to clean the dishes, but because I've told him so many little stories about my control issues from the past.

Now I'm forty, and it's so much easier to look back and see the source of my issues. I smile at having had such control issues and that I've spent over half my life trying to control my skin. Now, of course, that control has a very different face. It is one that is accepting and helps me discover new things and pushes me on this journey to help others take control of their health, and that is a good thing!

I now know that so many of my issues stem from feeling a lack of self-worth growing up. I didn't feel like enough, so looking back I'm not surprised at all that I got Ps. It has actually taught me that I am enough. The question is, how deep do we each need to go into our childhoods to find the source of our issues? I got a bit bullied, was crazy skinny when I was young, was looking for love in all the wrong places. I just needed love, and I think my family was so dysfunctional I didn't get enough of it.

Yes, my parents loved my siblings and me very much in their own way, did the best they could — heck, they raised us, and we are all okay and healthy and successful, so we turned out well. No drug addicts, as they would say. My dad was sick with his addiction, my mom was always scared, trying to raise us, being broke, etc. I got love, but maybe not as much as I needed back then. Maybe instead of my giving love to them in their hard times, they should have been giving more of it to me. Maybe this feeling of not being enough stemmed from that time in my life. Maybe you have been through a similar situation. Maybe my sharing this will give you the courage to go back and take a look.

I believe all of our issues stem from our childhood. Beliefs are ingrained in us without our even knowing. Being aware of what they are and where they come from is key. If you are aware, you can work on them a little each day. It's not easy, but it could help clear your skin and make you a much healthier and emotionally stable being.

My journey has taken me down some different and revealing paths, and I guess there was a reason I didn't have thick skin back when I was a child and in college. If I had, life would have handed me an entirely different set of obstacles, and I would never be here helping others. Strange how life turns out, as if it has a mind of its own, egging us to move on to what will really satisfy our soul versus what will just make us rich or famous because we think that's what we need to be a valuable person. I won't turn that option away, though, because that means I'm helping and getting to more and more suffering people out there, and making change. After all, as Gandhi said, "Be the change that you wish to see in the world."

Ps: My dad has been sober for over twenty years!

Meditation

One thing I've learned through years of therapy is that you cannot be truly happy while needing to be in complete control. It's just not possible, even if we convince ourselves otherwise. I want you to think about that as much as you can, because I see a common thread in many Ps sufferers and this is one of them.

I worked very hard on my issues over the years, but they still pop up here and there; so, don't give up, and know that we are all works-in-progress. When the control issues or fears come up, it's normal to think, "Really? Are you still here? I thought I got rid of you!"

For this exercise, I want you to think of one issue of yours that you feel is always lurking and holding you back from complete bliss. Thank it for coming into your life to teach you something important. Let go of needing to know what that reason is. Just know and believe that the reason will help bring you to your journey and that journey was meant to be lived by you, to bring you closer to your bliss. Don't sweat it, don't fear it, just work on it.

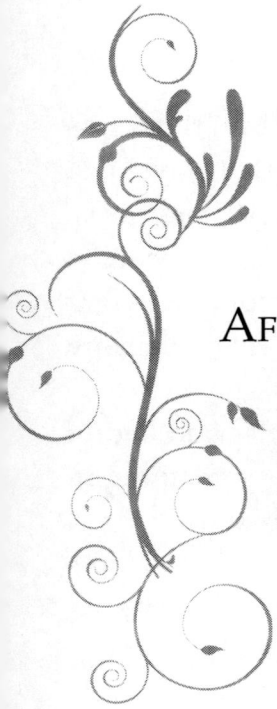

Just When I Thought I Had It Covered: My Accident

Since you cannot do good to all, you are to pay special attention to those who, by the accidents of time, or place, or circumstances, are brought into closer connection with you.

Augustine of Hippo

In the summer of 2013, a year and a half into being Ps clear, I had a terrible accident that turned my alkaline wagon upside down. I was working in TV at the time, and had gone to a nearby café to grab something for lunch. On my way down the aisle to the cashier, I passed a large bin of fresh smoothies and juices that were packed with ice. It was so packed that some of the ice had trickled out onto the floor, which was, unfortunately, a constant issue for them. I always saw people mopping it up and placing wet floor signs there. I never understood why they didn't just build a better bin or at least pack it less. There was such a simple solution. (My friend was in there recently and told me they still operate that way! I just hope other people don't experience what I did.) There I was, walking down the aisle and, before I could think, I slipped on ice and went down quickly with my legs in a split. My right leg went straight down in front of me without my having any control.

Now, I'm flexible, but I was in my late thirties and hadn't been able to do splits since my twenties. I felt something in my thigh stretch and rip or tear. That's the best way I can describe it. I was in utter pain and hysterically crying. People were gathered around me trying to help, but I felt paralyzed and couldn't move off the floor. All I felt was pain, and I knew something was terribly wrong. A worker there eventually managed to get me up off the floor onto a chair, but I wasn't able to sit in a normal position. I sort of lay on my side, holding on for dear life as the slightest movement caused severe pain throughout my leg. The café called my boss, and she rushed over with a few of my co-workers. We all sat there contemplating whether or not they should call an ambulance. I was hoping the pain would subside after some time, but it only got worse.

An ambulance took me to the hospital, where I was given pain medication and told by multiple doctors it was just a strain and that it would heal in time. I was instructed to leave on crutches and continue taking the pain medication and get lots of rest. Let me just explain something here: I was in so much pain that I was literally punching the bed. I felt nauseous because it was too much pain for me to handle. When they said it was a strain, everything in me knew it couldn't be just that. I told my boss how I felt, and she advised me to call my regular doctor as soon as I could to get an MRI. The hospital couldn't take X-rays that day because my leg was so inflamed and swollen that it was double the size of my other leg. It just wouldn't have been able to show a break or tear, which is what I assumed it had to have been. My mom and aunt drove into the city from Long Island to bring me home, which was a very rough ride. Living in the city on crutches is probably one of the hardest things I've ever done in my life. Even just getting into my apartment building up and down a few steps to the elevator was difficult. I wonder how people who are injured live in a walk up. Two weeks passed before I was able to get into a car service to go to see my doctor and get an MRI. It was the hardest two weeks to get through. I was on crutches, hobbling around my studio, unable to cook or go anywhere. I could barely pee in the toilet. Don't even ask me about my number two situation.

So finally, I was at my doctor's office bent over with my pants down. Fun! My pain was all along the back of my upper leg area. By this time the inflammation had gone down, but the back of my leg was black and blue from internal bleeding. My doctor took one look, was startled and said, "This is much worse than I thought. This was a pretty severe fall." So, off I went for an MRI.

I'll never forget that call with the results almost a week later. I was back at work, cabbing it back and forth because, even though I was off the crutches, I was still in pain while healing and couldn't walk up and down the subway steps. I had just stepped out of the car with my boss when my phone rang. My doctor said, "Kim, I'm shaking my head right now at your MRI results. It's way worse than I thought. Three of your hamstring tendons have ripped off of your pelvic bone, and you need surgery, ASAP." I didn't hear everything he said after that because I got very emotional and started crying. I handed the phone over to my boss and she got all the details from him.

Let me point out something here. While laid up at home this entire three weeks waiting for the inflammation to go down to get my MRI, I couldn't food shop, let alone cook. My mom and Mike came over to take care of me and feed me, but I pretty much ate what was convenient for them to make. Grilled cheese, chips, more grilled cheese, and canned soup. Mike did make me a big pot of homemade chicken soup after my surgery, but that was probably the healthiest I ate during that entire time. I'm pretty sure we got take-out a lot during that time. I wasn't complaining about it either because eating healthily was the last thing on my mind. I was too busy feeling depressed, which was such a foreign feeling to me. I'm naturally a very happy person, and sadness doesn't sit well with me. It sucked to be lying in bed all day, not able to move enough to take care of myself or even my dog. I'm not comfortable relying on others; I'm very independent and need to be up and about. It was torture for me to have no choice but to lie there until my body was healed enough to return to work. On top of that, Mike and I were pretty new, having been dating for only a few months. I knew we were falling in love, but I was nervous he would grow bored, or disenchanted. I couldn't leave my apartment. Somewhere in me, I was scared and insecure. As it turned out, this ended up bringing our relationship closer, but I wanted to point out all that was going on inside of me at the time: fear, anger, depression, and helplessness. Of course, I wasn't making it a point to eat healthfully. How can you, when you are not feeling good about yourself or your circumstances? And in this case, I truly had no control.

I finally had surgery a month later. They sewed my three hamstring tendons back onto my pelvic bone. I know, makes you cringe, right? I can't even believe I was walking around the city on one tendon for a month. The recovery period was that entire next year. That's a long time to be off the alkaline wagon. I ate healthy here and there, but there was something going on in me that made me sort of not care. A lot of effort goes into eating healthfully, and I just didn't have the drive to do it. I was working so hard, going to physical therapy three times a week while working full time, all while on crutches, and I think, somewhere deep down, I felt I deserved to eat whatever I wanted. I also didn't want to think about it.

So, of course, my Ps reared its ugly head, which only made me more depressed. After all the hard work I'd done on my journey clearing my skin, it felt like all it took was a bunch of pain medication (which has too many toxic reactions to list here), and processed food, and a negative state of mind for it to return. It came back too easily and too quickly, or so it felt. Looking back, I feel like the universe sent it back my way as a reminder to continue to love and take care of myself, but I didn't see it this way then. All I saw were two huge obstacles in front of me: to get my body back to where it was and to clear my skin *again*.

I couldn't shake that feeling of being defeated. I couldn't get out of my slump. Here I was making amazing strides in my therapy each week, getting a little stronger with each and every visit. At the same time, I was struggling with this feeling of failure. So on one level I was loving myself, taking care of my body the way I needed to, but I wasn't focused on the positive as much as the negative. My Ps was looking me in the face saying, "I'm baaaack. You thought you were rid of me. Guess again."

That year, giving in and allowing Ps to yet again have control over me because I lost my motivation and enthusiasm, all I had learned and applied in the past went out with it. What's crazy is that I knew deep down that I was the one in control, and I could heal my skin anytime I wanted. I knew what to do and could do it whenever I was ready. The problem was that I wasn't ready. I wasn't ready emotionally and I had a hard time trying to understand that. On one level, I couldn't handle the return of my Ps, but on another, I lacked the desire to do anything about it. There was a whole mental game that was going on in me and it was messing with my emotional state. I was back to that "Why me?" mentality, even though I knew better. I didn't need to be in that state, but I couldn't love myself enough to escape it. I tried so hard to be gentle with myself. I would get advice from family and friends who would say things like, "This is a tough journey for you right now; just focus on getting better." It would help me in the moment, but I had a hard time keeping that momentum going.

I see now I was beating myself up when what I needed to do was accept where I was at. Accepting where I was at was not in sight. At that time, my body needed me to show it love and all I was doing was showing it anger, resentment, and guilt. I was completely focused on the fact that it was all my fault that my Ps had returned. I let it happen. *Who cares that I had a traumatic experience and was in a year-long recovery program? What the heck is wrong with me?* My Ps had me judging myself so freaking harshly again. I didn't want to live a life like that, I thought.

Then, the turning point: Somehow I got angry at the Ps and that empowered the heck out of me. That was a good day. Finally, I was ready to get back on my alkaline wagon—and that's when my second journey began!

Everything I read about toxins in our system coming out in the form of Ps swam in my head. I took medications for about a month and absolutely noticed a difference. My elbows felt harder, rougher, thicker, and I was the walking example of what not to do if you suffer from Ps. But finally, I hit the wall and was ready.

You know that feeling, right? You know what you need to do, but don't want to do it. That could be related to every single thing in life, a job, a breakup, putting a pet down, an apology, taking responsibility for our bodies—the list goes on. What happens if you don't do it? There are negative consequences, usually. I just wanted to find a happy medium! That's all. If I could eat my favorite foods like buffalo wings and pizza, and if I could drink alcohol once or twice a week, I could deal with some dry skin. The key words here are dry and some. But for me, it's not dry and some, it was Ps patches in places that the world could see, and it made me feel ugly and ashamed again.

For most of us when we hit rock bottom, there arises the "eureka" moment that tells you it is time to start again because things are only going downhill quickly. My physical therapist always stresses the words "baby steps." I now find myself saying them in my head when I fall off the wagon, and I hope you remember to chant these words yourself when you need to: baby steps, baby steps, baby steps. Isn't that the way everything is in life or should be? Everything we experience has to start somewhere—whether it be love, work, health, or whatever, it's baby steps. I'll have only one glass of wine this weekend; baby steps. I will take a Dead Sea salt bath one day this week; baby steps. I will incorporate veggies into at least two of my meals today; baby steps. That's enough for this week! Go, me! What's enough for you?

I am sharing my terrible accident story in hopes this will convince you it is time. How about today you take the plunge and declare you are better than all of this and that you can be healed? Let the terrible experiences of the past, like my accident and falling off the wagon, bring you to a better point to realize your dream, just as I am now. Isn't it time that you created a closer connection to the most important person ever — you? I know you are worth it!

The following is a blog I wrote that I want to share here so that you can see how much passion I truly have for wanting to remain healed and for wanting to heal you:

Why I Want to Help People Heal and Love Their Skin[35]

I find it fascinating how the universe always seems to swoop in to reassure us when we are feeling fear about something we were born to do. Let me explain. I'm almost six months into my studies at the Institute for Integrative Nutrition to become a health coach, and I'm beyond scared! My passion is to specialize in helping people who suffer from skin diseases so I can help them heal the way I am healing myself, through nutrition and self-love. I'll be pre-certified in two weeks and have officially started my business, Healing My Skin. It's scary to start a new career at almost forty,

---

35   https://healingmypsoriasis.wordpress.com/2016/02/13/why-i-want-to-help-people-heal-love-their-skin/ (posted February 13, 2016).

and it doesn't help when the little voice in my head is negatively thinking thoughts like "What if I disappoint my clients?" Luckily, my passion and enthusiasm are keeping my negative thoughts at bay, and I'm not allowing fear to stop me. I genuinely love helping people, because it makes me feel so damn good inside, and I believe when you're passionate about something, you have to do it! Plus, everything in me believes in the healing power of whole foods and love, and my mission is to spread the word one person at a time!

I have been talking to a few people lately whom I consider to be my "practice clients." Some have psoriasis, and some just want to feel better in general. It's truly an honor to be on their journey! One of these practice clients, whom I now consider a friend, is a woman who has been suffering from severe psoriasis for a long time. She's a busy wife and mother of two little boys. When we first spoke, she admitted to being really nervous talking about her skin because, much like I had been when I was younger, she didn't talk to anyone about it, not even her husband. She hid it from most of the world as much as she could like a dirty little secret, feeling ashamed and embarrassed. She was disgusted by it, and when she found the courage to send me photos, I understood her fear.

This disease isn't pretty, but it's our bodies communicating with us that something needs to change. It took me over twenty years to listen, and I don't want others to have to wait that long. Can you imagine walking around feeling ashamed of your body every day of your life? We are not here to carry around feelings of shame and embarrassment; we are here to feel happiness and joy. At least, that's what I believe in every core of my being. It's why I finally "came out" about my psoriasis.

This woman I'm now friends with is so gorgeous, too— downright stunning! What's a shame is that someone so beautiful on both the inside and outside ended up feeling such disgust about herself. It makes me sad. I totally relate to what she has been feeling most of her life, which is what drives me to help people like her find their empowerment. In that empowerment, they find love and appreciation for themselves and their bodies. This beautiful woman started learning what was actually occurring inside of her body, how hard it was working to protect her, and she found a whole new respect and understanding for it. This changed everything for her, and she is starting to feel some control. She's not just looking at the symptom anymore; she's now looking at the cause.

This is what we all need to do with any illness or condition. We need to ask the question: What's causing this, and how can we work on healing that from the inside out? A perfect example is that when I get sick, it's always at a time when I'm most stressed out. My body is fighting to rest, and I'm usually not allowing it to. Then I get sick and am forced to cancel plans, not go to work, and lie on the couch.

This woman has been so inspired to heal, that in just one month, she has implemented new lifestyle changes into her family's home—which I'm sure wasn't easy, given that she has three boys! She sends me photos of her healthy cooking all the time, and I am so proud of her for staying motivated. I love getting those photos because I know she is now feeling the way I was feeling at the very beginning of my journey: open, hopeful, and excited. I am so happy for her that she feels in control of her body for the first time and ultimately feels more confident.

To see the changes in her skin only a month and a half into her new diet and her new outlook on life leaves me feeling elated. The feeling is enough to move mountains, people! It's A-mazing!

Our bodies are miracles, aren't they?

On the day she sent me some photos of her progress, they came with a beautiful message thanking me, telling me how grateful she was for having met me, that she and her husband both saw the difference and were so happy to see some clearing for the first time. Her text brought me to tears, because what she didn't know was that I was having such a bad day at work that day. I needed that text so badly. I was feeling no enjoyment in my day job anymore, on top of feeling doubt and fear about my new path as a health coach. The discouragement had me close to tears—then, bam! I got her text. I quietly thanked the universe because I knew, at that moment, it was reminding me that my path of true fulfillment was just starting. I smiled and thought, *I am meant to do this*. I believe everyone comes into our lives for a reason, no matter how big or small. She and I were so clearly meant to give each other empowerment, hope, confidence, and love—which heals a lot more than just our skin.

When you are having doubts about something in life, just ask the universe to show you the signs. It will, whether you want it to or not. Soon, with a positive attitude, your situation will change for the better or show you a new direction.

And, that is why healing Ps is all about love!

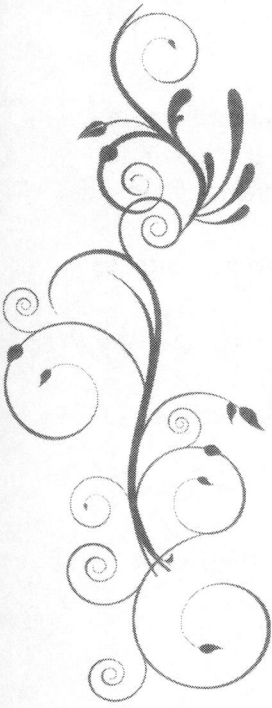

Bibliography

Resources & Cited Works

Axe, Dr. Josh. "4 Steps to Heal Leaky Gut and Autoimmune Disease." Dr. Axe. http://draxe.com/4-steps-to-heal-leaky-gut-and-autoimmune-disease/.

Ballantyne, Dr. Sarah. "The WHYs behind the Autoimmune Protocol: Nightshades." The Paleo Mom, August 22, 2012. http://www.thepaleomom.com/the-whys-behind-autoimmune-protocol/.

Barker, Leslie. "Psoriasis Research, Treatment Is Doctor's Life's Work." *The Charleston Gazette (Charleston, WV)*, November 27, 2012.

Cargill, Marie. *Acupuncture: A Viable Medical Alternative.* Westport, CT: Praeger Publishers, 1994.

Carr, Kris. *Crazy Sexy Diet: Eat Your Veggies, Ignite Your Spark, And Live Like You Mean It!* Skirt! Books, 2011.

"Cilantro Helped with Rash." *The Buffalo News (Buffalo, NY)*, May 5, 2014.

Clarke, Alex. "Chapter 2: The Challenges Facing Researchers in the Area." In *The Psychology of Appearance*, by Nichola Rumsey and Diana Harcourt, 28-62. Maidenhead, England: Open University Press, 2005.

"The Clean Fifteen." The Environmental Working Group. https://www.ewg.org/foodnews/clean_fifteen_list.php.

Cove, Julie. "Alkaline Foods Chart." Alkaline Sisters (blog). http://www.alkalinesisters.com/alkaline-food-chart/.

Deutsch, Jelix. *Body, Mind, and the Sensory Gateways*. New York: Basic Books, 1963.

"The Dirty Dozen." The Environmental Working Group. https://www.ewg.org/foodnews/dirty_dozen_list.php.

Ede, Dr. Georgia. "How Deadly Are Nightshades?" Diagnosis Diet. http://www.diagnosisdiet.com/nightshades/.

Flanagan, Caitlin. "The Kingdoms of Narcissism." *International New York Times*, September 3, 2015.

Fonseca, Jose. *Contemporary Psychodrama: New Approaches to Theory and Technique*. New York: Brunner-Routledge, 2004.

Fuhrman, Joel. *Eat to Live: The Revolutionary Formula for Fast and Sustained Weight Loss*. Little, Brown and Company, 2005.

Germer, Christopher K., Ronald D. Siegel, and Paul R. Fulton, eds. *Mindfulness and Psychotherapy*. New York: Guilford Press, 2005.

Goldhirsch, Dr. Mark. "Nutrition Response Testing." Dr. Mark Goldhirsch Chiropractic & Nutrition. http://drmarkg.com/nutrition/nutrition-response-testing.html.

Gunnars, Kris, "11 Proven Health Benefits of Chia Seeds," Authority Nutrition, https://authoritynutrition.com/11-proven-health-benefits-of-chia-seeds/.

Hay, Louise. *Heal Your Body: The Mental Causes for Physical Illness and the Metaphysical Way to Overcome Them*. Carlsbad, CA: Hay House, 1988.

Hay, Louise. "Mirror, Mirror, on the Wall…" Heal Your Life (blog), October 26, 2009, http://www.healyourlife.com/mirror-mirror-on-the-wall.

Hari, Vani. The Food Babe (blog), http://foodbabe.com/.

Hofmekler, Ori. Hyman, "Vitamin Poisoning: Are We Destroying Our Health with Hi-Potency Synthetic Vitamins?" Organic Consumer's Association, https://www.organicconsumers. org/news/vitamin-poisoning-are-we-destroying-our-health-hi-potency-synthetic-vitamins.

Hyman, Dr. Mark. "10 Steps to Reverse Autoimmune Disease," Dr. Hyman (blog), September 4, 2015, http://drhyman.com/blog/2015/09/04/10-steps-to-reverse-autoimmune-disease/.

"A Gut Feeling." *Daily Herald (Arlington Heights, IL)*, October 28, 2013.

Jacoby, David B., and Robert M. Youngson. *Encyclopedia of Family Health*. 3rd ed. Vol. 12. New York: Marshall Cavendish, 2005.

King, John E., ed. *Mayo Clinic on Digestive Health*. Philadelphia: Mason Crest, 2002.

Klein, Norman, ed. *Culture, Curers, and Contagion: Readings for Medical Social Science*. Novato, CA: Chandler and Sharp, 1979.

Komaroff, Anthony. "Effects of Psoriasis Are Not Confined to the Skin." *Pittsburgh Post-Gazette (Pittsburgh, PA)*, October 7, 2014.

Lakshmy, Sreelatha, Sivaprakash Balasundaram, Sukanto Sarkar, Moutusi Audhya, and Eswaran Subramaniam. "A Cross-Sectional Study of Prevalence and Implications of Depression and Anxiety in Psoriasis." *Indian Journal of Psychological Medicine* 37, no. 4 (2015).

Lawrence, Glen D. *The Fats of Life: Essential Fatty Acids in Health and Disease*. New Brunswick, NJ: Rutgers University Press, 2010.

"Learn to Love the Skin You're In. HEALTH How Your Pharmacist Can Help You Manage Your Common Skin Conditions." *The Mirror (London, England)*, December 8, 2015.

Lorand, Sandor, ed. *Psychoanalysis Today*. New York: International University Press, 1944.

Maciocia, Giovanni. *The Foundations of Chinese Medicine: A Comprehensive Text for Acupuncturists and Herbalists*. Edinburgh: Churchill Livingstone, 1989.

Mielke, James H., Lyle W. Konigsberg, and John H. Relethford. *Human Biological Variation*. New York: Oxford University Press, 2006.

Norman, Robert A. *The Woman Who Lost Her Skin: (And Other Dermatological Tales)*. New York: Routledge, 2004.

Nutton, Vivian. *Ancient Medicine*. London: Routledge, 2004.

Ogden, Jane. *Health Psychology: A Textbook*. 4th ed. Maidenhead, England: Open University Press, 2007.

O'Neill, Barbara. "Acid Alkaline Balance." May 17, 2012, https://youtu.be/BBl1QDag2-8.

Pagano, Dr. John O. A. *Healing Psoriasis: The Natural Alternative* Hoboken, NJ: John Wiley & Sons; 2008.

"The PS5 Oat Cream That Celebrities Swear By." *Daily Mail (London)*, March 31, 2016.

Ringwald, Christopher D. *The Soul of Recovery: Uncovering the Spiritual Dimension in the Treatment of Addictions*. New York: Oxford University Press, 2002.

Roberts, Jane. *The Way Toward Health: A Seth Book*. Amber-Allen, 1997.

Sathyanarayana Rao, T. S; Basavaraj, K.H.; and Das, Keya. "Psychosomatic paradigms in psoriasis: Psoriasis, stress and mental health," *Indian Journal of Psychiatry*, 2013 Oct-Dec; 55(4). 313–315.

Scambler, Graham, ed. *Habermas, Critical Theory and Health*. London: Routledge, 2001.

Schalock, Dr. Peter C. "Psoriasis," Merck Manual, http://www.merckmanuals.com/professional/dermatologic-disorders/psoriasis-and-scaling-diseases/psoriasis.

Sherman, Carl. "Depression, Dissected." *Psychology Today*, July/August 2015, 33+.

Silverstone, Alicia. *The Kind Diet*. New York: Rodale, 2009.

"Sometimes Politeness Is a Curse." *Liverpool Echo (Liverpool, England)*, October 11, 2015.

Strom, Charles M. *Heredity and Ability: How Genetics Affects Your Child and What You Can Do about It*. New York: Plenum Press, 1990.

"This Celebrity Favourite Is Worth Its Salt; They Have Been Used
    for Centuries for Their Therapeutic Benefits, and They're
    Still Popular with Athletes to Aid Muscle Recovery. Abi
    Jackson Learns of the Wonders of Humble Bath Salts."
    Western Mail (Cardiff, Wales), May 19, 2014.
Van Der Steen, Wim J., Vincent K.Y Ho, and Ferry J. Karmelk.
    *Beyond Boundaries of Biomedicine: Pragmatic
    Perspectives on Health and Disease*. At the Interface/
    Probing the Boundaries. Amsterdam: Rodopi, 2003.
Walker, Ruth. "Spot the Difference." *Scotland on Sunday
    (Edinburgh, Scotland)*, June 17, 2012.
"When an Itch Wrecks Your Life — and NOTHING Can Get Rid
    of It." *Daily Mail (London)*, April 8, 2014.
Zusne, Leonard, and Warren H. Jones. *Anomalistic Psychology: A
    Study of Magical Thinking*. 2nd ed. Hillsdale, NJ: Lawrence
    Erlbaum Associates, 1989.

Films

The Beautiful Truth: The World's Simplest Cure for Cancer,
    directed by Steve Kroschel (2008; Cinema Libre Studio).
Crazy Sexy Cancer, directed by Kris Carr (2008; Gaiam
    Entertainment).
Fat, Sick & Nearly Dead, directed by Joe Cross (2011; Passion
    River Films).
Food Inc., directed by Robert Kenner, written by Robert Kenner
    and Elise Pearlstein (2009; Magnolia Home Entertainment).
Food Matters, directed by James Colquhoun, Laurentine Ten
    Bosch (2009; Passion River Films).
The Gerson Miracle, directed by Steve Kroschel (2009; Cinema
    Libre Studio).
Hungry for Change, directed by James Colquhoun, Laurentine Ten
    Bosch, Carlo Ledesma (2012; Docurama).

CPSIA information can be obtained
at www.ICGtesting.com
Printed in the USA
FSOW01n0645180117
29765FS

9 781478 779247